Visual Agnosia

Issues in the Biology of Language and Cognition
John C. Marshall, editor

What the Hands Reveal about the Brain
Howard Poizner, Edward S. Klima, and Ursula Bellugi, 1987

Disorders of Syntactic Comprehension
David N. Caplan and Nancy Hildebrandt, 1987

Missing the Meaning? A Cognitive Neuropsychological Study of the Processing of Words by an Aphasic Patient
David Howard and Susan Franklin, 1988

The Psychobiology of Down Syndrome
edited by Lynn Nadel, 1988

From Reading to Neurons
edited by Albert M. Galaburda, 1989

Visual Agnosia: Disorders of Object Recognition and What They Tell Us About Normal Vision
Martha J. Farah, 1990

Theoretical Perspectives on Language Deficits
Yosef Grodzinsky, 1990

Modular Deficits in Alzheimer-Type Dementia
Myrna F. Schwartz, 1990

Laura: A Case Study for the Modularity of Language
Jeni Yamada, 1990

Visual Agnosia

Disorders of Object Recognition and What They Tell Us about Normal Vision

Martha J. Farah

A Bradford Book

The MIT Press
Cambridge, Massachusetts
London, England

Fourth printing, 1999

First MIT Press paperback edition, 1995
© 1990 Massachusetts Institute of Technology

This book was set in Palatino by The MIT Press. It was printed and bound in the United States of America.

Library of Congress Cataloging in Publication Data

Farah, Martha J.
    Visual agnosia: disorders of object recognition and what they tell us about normal vision / Martha J. Farah.
        p. cm—(Issues in the biology of language and cognition)
    "A Bradford book."
    Includes bibliographical references.
    ISBN 0-262-06135-X (HB), 0-262-56082-8 (PB)
    1. Visual agnosia. 2. Visual perception. I. Title. II. Series.
    [DNLM: 1. Agnosia—physiopathology. 2. Form Perception—physiology. WL 340 F219v]
    RC394.V57F37   1990
    617.7—dc20
    DNLM/DLC
for Library of Congress   89-14283
                                                                          CIP

To Hermine Makman

Contents

Foreword
Seeing, Knowing, and Believing
John C. Marshall

Chomsky (1968) has reflected that

> One difficulty in the psychological sciences lies in the familiarity of
> the phenomena with which they deal. A certain intellectual effort is
> required to see how such phenomena can pose serious problems or
> call for intricate explanatory theories. One is inclined to take them
> for granted as necessary or somehow "natural."

Nowhere, perhaps, is this familiarity more pernicious than in the study
of perception. The common man (or woman) would, it might be argued,
simply fail to see a problem: If, in good illumination (and wearing my
glasses), my eyes alight upon an everyday scene, then "I just see a table
with a cup on it some little distance to my left." End of story.

Such inquiry-stopping remarks are never, of course, actually uttered
by the man on the tram; rather, they are placed in his mouth by
professional philosophers. Thus Hamlyn (1957), for example, argues that
veridical perception needs no explanation; only the erroneous percept
demands an accounting. (Imagine this claim in any other area of biology:
Harvey was misguided to inquire into the structure and function of the
normal heart; only heart attacks require explanation.)

One counter to this strange view is, broadly speaking, computational:
Make me a formal model of how the mind-brain transforms peripheral
sensory transduction (the two-dimensional mosaic of retinal stimulation) into the full perceptual richness of three-dimensional objects in
space. That research program could keep experimental psychologists,
neurophysiologists, and workers in artificial intelligence busy for some
years (Marr 1982). And it would undoubtedly require us to understand
how I recognize a cat as a cat (before considering how, on occasion, I
might mistake one for a squirrel). However, even this enterprise has been
regarded as one of dubious validity. Searle (1984), for example, contrasts
the ease with which we recognize the faces of friends and relatives with
the complexity of the geometric and topologic calculations required to
simulate our ability in this domain. And he uses these premises to infer

that the brain may not, in any sense, *compute* facial identities. "When we step in wet sand and make a footprint," Searle writes, "neither our feet nor the sand does any computing." Yet "a program that would calculate the topology of a footprint from information about differential pressures on the sand . . . would be a fairly complex computational task." Whence Searle reaches the conclusion that facial recognition may be "as simple and as automatic as making footprints in the sand"! What can one say to someone who believes that faces (and footprints) are recognized *tout court* by virtue of the imprint that they leave in the brain? Only that Plato (in *Theaetetus*) was there first ("Suppose, then, I beg, for the sake of argument, that we have in our souls a waxen tablet. . . ."). And that the claims of more sophisticated theories of "direct perception" have been adequately disposed of by Fodor and Pylyshyn (1981).

Searle does at least concede that relatively discrete regions of the brain are selectively (and causally) implicated in visual recognition and, hence, that different physiological substrates are functionally specialized. But other philosophers have even managed to find the entire concept of an intelligible relationship between functional description and physical instantiation incoherent; they must, one presumes, repair their bicycles by trial-and-error. Thus Hacker (1987), for example, objects to the notion that cells in area V4 use information from the output of V1 "to assign colours to surfaces." The reason, it appears, is that neither cells nor collections thereof can be said to use information; the predicate is applicable, by fiat, only to the activities of a whole person (a concept that Hacker nowhere explicates).

Happily, these bizarre musings have not impeded the progress of cognitive neuropsychology at either an empirical or a theoretical level.

The language of information processing (more generally, of engineering) is thus far the only language we have invented that maps between the flux of the external world and our mental representation thereof. To the best of our knowledge, such mentation does not exist in the absence of physical (physiological) instantiation. It thus follows that information-processing psychology is the only language in which we can formally describe what brains do at a level that goes significantly beyond discussion of, say, the firing rates of assemblies of neurons.

Perceptual psychology, conceived as the study of the assignment of structural descriptions to visual stimulation, has of course a long and illustrious history. Its first high point can be seen in the achievements of the gestalt psychologists from Köhler (1924) to Kanizsa (1979). On the basis of such work, combined now with the hard but necessary task of modeling explicitly how information can be extracted from images (Marr 1982), no scientist could imagine that vision is too "natural" to demand explanation.

However, in healthy condition, the visual system may operate too smoothly and seamlessly for us to grasp the modus operandi of its component parts. Thus, as with any other complex biological function, there is the strong possibility that brain damage, by rudely tearing apart and isolating the elements of an integrated mechanism, will throw light upon the structure of the normal system. It is here that pathology shocks us out of the complacency so acutely diagnosed by Chomsky (1968). Selective impairments in the perception of form (Campion and Latto 1985), color (Heywood, Wilson, and Cowey 1987), intensity (Stoerig 1987), orientation (Solms, Kaplan-Solms, Saling, and Miller 1988), and location in space (Marsh and Philwin 1987) virtually force one to consider how separate informational channels interact to provide an integrated visual world.

The discovery of conditions such as "blindsight" (Weiskrantz 1986), in which patients can (to a limited extent) "see" without "knowing" that they see, likewise forces a distinction of "processing levels" within the visual system. Blindsight, and related phenomena of "tacit knowledge" (de Haan, Young, and Newcombe 1987; Marshall and Halligan 1988) may eventually enable us to approach (some aspects of) consciousness within a genuinely biological context. Like all pathologies, these dissociations within the visual world make the natural surprising yet give rise to (scientific) problems, not pure mysteries. The value of familiarity with cognitive disorder can be seen across all the disciplines concerned with the understanding of human nature. During the 1920s, one of the most original and insightful German neurologists, Kurt Goldstein, used to take his cousin, an equally distinguished philosopher, on ward rounds at the Frankfurt Neurological Institute. The third volume of Ernst Cassirer's *Philosophy of Symbolic Forms* (1965; 1953-1957) shows clearly how Kantian metaphysics can be constrained and deepened by the empirical findings of behavioral neurology.

The presence of philosophers on ward rounds is still, unfortunately, rare, but experimental psychologists are rapidly becoming a crucial "resource." Martha Farah's work is located firmly and centrally in the tradition of modern neuropsychology: the combined study of normal and pathological cognition, interpreted within an information-processing framework. The specific topic of her book—*Visual Agnosia*—refers to a condition in which the patient fails to recognize objects (by sight) despite relatively well-preserved sensory capacities and no evidence of a more generalized dementia. In one form of the syndrome, the patient may be well able to describe verbally the characteristic form and function of, say, a chair; he or she also may be able to draw a chair from a model (real object or line drawing thereof) with sufficient accuracy so that we can recognize the identity of the copy. Yet despite these abilities, the patient cannot "see" that a chair is a chair is a chair.

As with all other taxonomic labels in behavioral neurology, visual agnosia covers a huge range of quite distinct conditions in which different components and processing levels are impaired within the visual system (and beyond). Farah's first major achievement in this book is to construct a fine-grained taxonomy that does justice to both clinical symptomatology and the anatomical loci of the responsible brain damage. More crucially, the taxonomy is rationally constrained by findings from perceptual experimentation with normal subjects and by models formulated in (computationally based) cognitive science.

As Farah herself notes, theories do not spring automatically from (even good) taxonomies. But at the very least this essential ground-clearing operation brings some meaningful order to over a century of clinical reports that have sometimes spread more confusion than enlightenment. Good theory presupposes that one can see the wood (in addition to the trees). And here, too, Farah conjectures a functional architecture for the object recognition (and naming) system that is sufficiently explicit to drive further empirical research and theoretical advance. The scope of the volume is wide; it covers, critically but fairly, category-specific deficits (including pure alexia and prosopagnosia) and modality-specific deficits (the optic aphasias) in addition to the full range of "apperceptive" and "associative" disorders of object recognition per se. The interaction of spatial attention and "memory" with recognition processes is emphasized. And throughout, hypothesized functional components of the system are linked to their neuroanatomic correlates.

Visual Agnosia will undoubtedly prove a seminal contribution to cognitive neuroscience.

References

Campion, J., and Latto, R. (1985). Apperceptive agnosia due to carbon monoxide poisoning. *Behavioral Brain Research* 15:227–240.

Cassirer, E. (1965). *The Philosophy of Symbolic Forms.* Vol. 3, *The Phenomenology of Knowledge* New Haven: Yale University Press.

Chomsky, N. (1968). *Language and Mind.* New York: Harcourt Brace Jovanovich.

de Haan, E. H. F., Young, A. W., and Newcombe, F. (1987). Face recognition without awareness. *Cognitive Neuropsychology* 4:385–415.

Fodor, J. A., and Pylyshyn, Z. W. (1981). How direct is visual perception? Some reflections on Gibson's "Ecological Approach." *Cognition* 9:139–196.

Hacker, P. (1987). Languages, minds and brains. In C. Blakemore and S. Greenfield, eds; *Mindwaves: Thoughts on Intelligence, Identity, and Consciousness.* Oxford: Basil Blackwell.

Hamlyn, D. (1957). *The Psychology of Perception.* London: Routledge and Kegan Paul.

Heywood, C. A., Wilson, B., and Cowey, A. (1987). A case study of cortical colour 'blindness' with relatively intact achromatic discrimination. *Journal of Neurology, Neurosurgery, and Psychiatry* 50:22–29.

Kanizsa, G. (1979). *Organization of Vision: Essays on Gestalt Perception*. New York: Praeger.

Köhler, W. (1924). The problem of form in perception. *British Journal of Psychology* 14:262–268.

Marr, D. (1982). *Vision*. San Francisco: Freeman.

Marsh, G. G., and Philwin, B. (1987). Unilateral neglect and constructional apraxia in a right-handed artist with a left posterior lesion. *Cortex* 23:149–155.

Marshall, J. C., and Halligan, P. W. (1988). Blindsight and insight in visuo-spatial neglect. *Nature* 336:766–767.

Searle, J. (1984). *Minds, Brains and Science*. London: British Broadcasting Corporation.

Solms, M., Kaplan-Solms, K., Saling, M., and Miller, P. (1988). Inverted vision after frontal lobe damage. *Cortex* 24:499–509.

Stoerig, P. (1987). Chromaticity and achromaticity: Evidence for a functional differentiation in visual field deficits. *Brain* 110:869–886.

Weiskrantz, L. (1986). *Blindsight: A Case Study and Implications*. Oxford: Clarendon.

Preface

A couple of years ago I began reading the neuropsychology literature on disorders of visual object recognition. Although my initial motivation was to try to learn more about mental imagery, as higher levels of visual representation seem to be shared by both imagery and perception, I soon found the agnosia literature quite fascinating in its own right. Unfortunately, I also found it quite confusing. For one thing, the data themselves are messy: There is a vast array of abilities and deficits associated with any given patient, and no two patients are identical. Different writers focus on different aspects of these data, and as a result the same patient is sometimes cited by different writers as an example of different syndromes—conceptually distinct and occasionally even mutually exclusive syndromes! In addition, relatively little work has been done relating agnosia to current conceptions of visual object recognition in cognitive science, the field in which I feel most at home. Therefore, the questions and assumptions behind the case reports, not to mention their terminology, were quite foreign to me.

In the end I spent the better part of a year just reading case reports and trying to get a feel for the patterns in the data. Chapters 2 and 4 reflect the outcome of this process. In these chapters I propose groupings of cases using as purely empirical, "bottom-up" criteria as possible. In some instances these groupings are not so radically different from those of other writers, but in others they do involve subdividing or merging standard taxonomic categories to better capture the patterns of similarities and differences among the cases. Of course, taxonomies are only of interest insofar as they organize the data base for purposes of developing and testing theories. That is the real goal of this book.

A valid taxonomy is a necessary condition for theoretical progress, but not a sufficient one. It would be naive to think that, if the data are only arranged in the right way, a Theory will come bounding out at the observer. What the neuropsychological data do yield are clues, constraints, pieces of a puzzle that show some encouraging signs of fitting together with our understanding of object recognition from other fields: cognitive psychology, neurophysiology, and computational vision. In chapters 3, 5, and 6 I attempt to interpret the different agnosic syndromes in terms of theories of normal object recognition, and to derive constraints on those theories from the phenomena of agnosia.

There are many people who contributed, directly or indirectly, to this book. Clark Glymour, John Marshall, Steven Pinker, Robin Rochlin, Marcie Wallace, and an anonymous reviewer read the entire manuscript and gave many insightful comments and suggestions. David Plaut read the sections on connectionism and helped make these sections clearer and more accurate. Fiona Stevens at the MIT Press was as encouraging and supportive as she was knowledgeable and efficient; it was a lucky day for me when I decided to call publishers and started (and stopped!) with Fiona. Karen Klein and Robin Rochlin tracked down and xeroxed scores of references each, and Muriel Fleishman and Kim Murray provided skilled secretarial help. Less tangible, but no less important, are the insights and encouragement I have received over the past few years from many teachers and collaborators in the areas of neuropsychology and visual cognition. In graduate school, I worked first with Stephen Kosslyn and then with R. Duncan Luce, two excellent advisors who supplied me with a many-sided education. As a postdoctoral fellow I was advised by both Howard Gardner and Steven Pinker, who continued to offer me a broad and eclectic view of the field, as well as the benefit of their tremendous knowledge of neuropsychology and visual cognition. During these and subsequent years I also had the privilege of working with some outstanding clinician-scientists, including Ron Calvanio, David Levine, and Graham Ratcliff, who patiently waited out my delusion that all neuropsychological phenomena must be simple deletions of a cognitive psychologist's preconceived box or arrow, and showed me how much more can be learned from the careful and truly open-minded examination of people with brain damage. From Franck Peronnet and his colleagues at INSERM Unit 280 in Lyon I learned much about visual electrophysiology, the French language (invaluable for reading the many case reports in that language), and food, wine, and travel (invaluable when I'd read too many case reports). For the past four years Harold Goodglass has generously included me in the Aphasia Research Center of the Boston University School of Medicine, making Boston my home away from home, as well as a much appreciated source of intellectual and financial support. I also owe a debt of thanks to my colleagues at Carnegie-Mellon, who made the dreaded assistant professor years a stimulating and enjoyable time in my life, and the funding agencies who have generously supported my research and writing, the National Institutes of Health, the Office of Naval Research, and the Alfred P. Sloan Foundation. Finally, I thank my parents, Helen and Ted Farah, for their support and encouragement throughout my education and career.

Visual Agnosia

Chapter 1
Introduction

Brain damage can lead to relatively selective impairments in language, memory, attention, motor skills, or vision. One of the reasons for studying the cognitive impairments that follow brain damage is for the clues they can give us about normal cognition. By studying the way in which a system breaks down, we can put constraints on how it was organized in the first place. Reciprocally, the study of normal cognition can aid our understanding of cognitive disorders. To go beyond the superficial characterization of a cognitive disorder in terms of tests that a patient can and cannot perform, to a characterization of the disorder in terms of the underlying components of the cognitive architecture that have been damaged, we must have a theory of what the components of the cognitive architecture are and how they are used in performing the relevant tests. The explicit goal of the new field of "cognitive neuropsychology" is to relate models of normal cognition to neuropsychological phenomena, for the purpose of advancing our understanding of cognition in both normal and brain-damaged people.

Impairment in the higher visual processes necessary for object recognition, with relative preservation of elementary visual functions, is known as visual agnosia. The exact nature of the preserved and impaired visual capabilities can vary considerably from one agnosic patient to another. Specific cases will be described in detail in subsequent chapters, but a few examples will be mentioned here to give the reader a sense of the range of the phenomena from the outset. Some agnosic patients cannot recognize common objects even though they can see them well enough to draw accurate copies of them. For example, a patient described by Rubens and Benson (1971) was unable to identify any of the drawings shown in figure 1, despite his perfectly recognizable copies of them. He refused to try to name the key, said the pig "could be a dog or any other animal," the bird "could be a beech stump," and the train "a wagon or car of some kind; the larger vehicle is being pulled by the smaller one" (p. 310). The difficulty is not limited to the naming of objects; it is equally present when nonverbal tests of recognition are used, such as pantomiming the use of an object, or sorting objects into groups

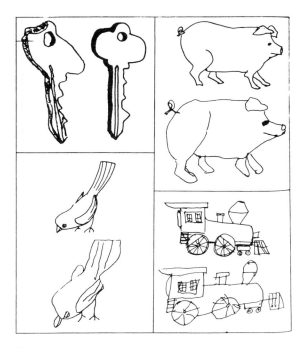

Figure 1
Three drawings and the copies made by the associative agnosic patient studied by Rubens and Benson (1971). Despite being able to see the drawings well enough to copy them, the patient was unable to recognize them.

according to semantic association strength or similarity of function. Nor is the difficulty attributable to a general loss of knowledge about objects, as these patients can readily identify objects by their characteristic sounds, or by their feel when touched. In other agnosic patients, the recognition impairment may be broader or narrower in scope. For example, some patients cannot even recognize simple forms such as a circle or a square, despite adequate acuity and the ability to trace the complete form with their fingers (e.g., Benson and Greenberg, 1969). Other patients can recognize most objects and encounter difficulty mainly with faces (e.g., Pallis, 1955), sometimes to the point of being unable to recognize members of their own family, or even their own face in a mirror.

1.1 A Brief History of Agnosia

Object recognition and the agnosias have been a rather neglected subject in cognitive neuropsychology. One measure of this can be gleaned from the tables of contents of journals: Studies of aphasics, alexics, and amnesics dominate the cognitively-oriented neuropsychology journals, as well as making an occasional appearance in cognitive psychology journals. In contrast, one reads much less about disorders of visual object recognition in general, and very little that speaks directly to issues and theories in cognitive science. This is partly attributable to the history of cognitive science itself: It has, until recently, been dominated by the study of verbal thinking and memory, topics which seemed particularly compatible with the conception of the mind as a symbol-manipulating computer. Comprehensive theories in the domain of visual cognition are new in cognitive psychology, as is apparent from the publication dates of such "classic" writings as Marr (1982) and Biederman (1987) on visual object recognition, Posner (1980) and Triesman and Gelade (1980) on visual attention, and Kosslyn (1980) and Shepard (1978) on visual imagery. Not surprisingly, then, it is only very recently that cognitive neuropsychologists have been able to use these theoretical developments in their analysis of higher visual disorders.

In the cognitive neuropsychology of visual object recognition, progress has been constrained not only by a general dearth of theory in visual cognition, but also by the extreme rarity of the relevant syndrome, visual agnosia. Agnosia is sufficiently rare that, until recently, its very existence has been an issue of contention! First Bay (1953), and then Bender and Feldman (1972) argued that visual agnosia, in the sense of a selective impairment in visual recognition per se, does not exist. Bay proposed that the appearance of a selective impairment in object recognition was invariably the result of a combination of two more general characteristics of agnosic patients: First, he suggested that these patients always have subtle impairments in elementary visual functions, which may be less apparent under the conditions of standard tests of visual fields, acuity, etc., than when they are being used for object recognition under natural conditions. Second, he claimed that these patients suffer from a general intellectual decline. According to Bay, impairments in elementary vision and general intelligence may occasionally conspire to produce disproportionate difficulties with object recognition, but there is no such thing as an impairment in object recognition per se. Bender and Feldman (1972) supported Bay's claims with a systematic review of a large number of neurological patients: They searched all of the patient records from a twenty-year period at New York's Mount Sinai Hospital and found relatively few cases with visual recognition difficulties. What they took to be more damaging to the concept of agnosia was the fact that all of these cases also had some significant elementary visual and/or general intellectual impairments.

Bay, Bender, and Feldman won over many influential neuropsychologists to their point of view on agnosia (e.g., Critchley, 1964; Teuber, 1968), but their skepticism was not shared by everyone. Even though a "pure" case of agnosia (a patient with impaired visual object recognition and perfectly normal elementary visual and intellectual capabilities) would disprove the skeptics' position, the absence of such a case does not prove it. Neuropsychologists know far too well that "nature's experiments" are executed rather sloppily, and they would have very little to study if they confined themselves to pure cases of anything. With this in mind, Ettlinger (1956) made the important observation that finding a "pure" agnosic was not the only way to settle the issue empirically. Just as effective would be the demonstration that agnosic patients were no more impaired in their intellectual and elementary visual capabilities than many nonagnosic patients. He demonstrated that this was true by systematically assessing a variety of elementary visual functions in patients already screened for generalized intellectual decline. Although only one of his cases had a true agnosia, and this case did have elementary visual impairments, he found other patients with more severe elementary visual impairments who were not agnosic.

Contemporary readers may be puzzled by the level of skepticism directed at the concept of agnosia. Why the impulse to try to "explain away" agnosia, but not, say, aphasia? One could imagine a similar argument being made that nonfluent aphasia represents a combination of dysarthria and general cognitive decline, and yet such arguments were not made. The explanation may lie in the conceptions of normal visual object recognition that were prevalent at the time. If one views object recognition as taking place in two relatively undifferentiated stages, namely (1) seeing the object and (2) associating general knowledge of the object with the percept, then the only possible way to disrupt object recognition is by disrupting vision or general knowledge. If object recognition difficulties seem disproportionate to difficulties of vision or general knowledge (as is the case, by definition, with visual agnosia), then this must be due to a synergistic interaction of minor difficulties in both vision and general knowledge. In contrast, if one views object recognition as involving a series of stimulus representations with increasingly greater abstraction from the retinal array and increasingly greater correspondence with invariant properties of objects in the physical world, as most current vision researchers do (e.g., Marr, 1982), then brain damage affecting just the later stages of vision could in principle create a "pure" visual agnosia. Bay's view of normal object recognition did, in fact, include only two kinds of representation, modality-specific elementary sensory representation and amodal higher-level knowledge representations. He excluded, a priori, the idea of higher level visual representations: "There is neither a [visual] gnostic function nor a specific disorder of this function. Such apparently gnostic activities . . . [are due to] sensory functions or to general psychological qualities which are not confined to a certain sensory sphere" (p.550).

One of the legacies of this controversy has been a rather cautious, descriptive approach to the study of agnosia. The goal of most case studies has been to document, as carefully as possible, that agnosia exists. This is accomplished by demonstrating an impairment in object recognition, and then assessing the patients' general intellectual abilities and elementary visual abilities, and showing them to be at least as good as those of many patients who do not have impairments in object recognition. The attempt to explain the phenomena of agnosia, or to relate them to questions about visual object recognition, has been made far less often. When such an attempt is made, the focus has generally been on traditional neuropsychological concerns such as localization (e.g., Albert, Soffer, Silverberg, and Reches, 1979), disconnection versus functional loss (e.g., Geschwind, 1965), and the delineation of syndromes (e.g., Bornstein and Kidron, 1959). Although exceptions exist (e.g., Ratcliff and Newcombe, 1982; Humphreys and Riddoch, 1987), there has been disappointingly little effort made to relate the phenomena of agnosia to current cognitive theories of object recognition. In the following chapters I will describe and interpret the different agnosic syndromes in terms of theories of normal vision, and I will bring these syndromes to bear as evidence on a variety of questions in the study of higher vision. For example, are there different recognition modules, or subsystems, required for recognizing different kinds of stimuli (e.g., faces, common objects, printed words)? Does visual selective attention operate prior to object recognition, subsequent to it, or in parallel with it? Are the long-term visual memory representations underlying recognition implemented locally or in a distributed network? Is the search process whereby a stimulus is matched with these representations more consistent with a computational architecture based on symbol manipulation or massively parallel constraint satisfaction?

1.2 Types of Agnosia

Taxonomizing may appear to be a rather atheoretical enterprise, which would be better replaced by analysis of the phenomena of agnosia using cognitive theories. However, we must begin with issues of taxonomy because grouping the phenomena correctly, in any area of science, is a prerequisite for making useful theoretical generalizations about them. This is all the more important—and all the more difficult—in the study of agnosia because the entire data base is comprised of single cases, no two of which are exactly alike. Therefore, the first order of business is to delineate different types of agnosia, which can then be interpreted in terms of damage to particular components of theories of object recognition, and which can also thereby constrain theories of object recognition.

There is no standard taxonomy of agnosia. Everyone agrees that agnosic patients differ from one another in certain ways, but the question of which differences are differences of degree and which are differences of kind has not found a unanimous answer. On careful reading of patients' abilities and deficits, I find that many authors have grouped patients in unhelpful ways. Their implicit taxonomies misrepresent the basic empirical phenomena, both by overinclusive categories that blur theoretically important distinctions between different syndromes, and by overfractionation of syndromes, in which differences of degree are treated as differences of kind. Therefore, the present discussion of agnosia will start with a taxonomy, the goal of which is to sort the phenomena out into their true "natural kinds." In chapters 2 and 4 I present this taxonomy, derived as much as possible from purely empirical considerations, that is, letting the natural category structure of the phenomena "speak for themselves" without the imposition of any theoretical ideas from me. Theoretical interpretations of these phenomena are segregated into separate chapters and presented after the data themselves.

Most neuropsychologists follow Lissauer (1890) in distinguishing between the "apperceptive agnosias" and the "associative agnosias." According to Lissauer, apperceptive agnosias are those in which recognition fails because of an impairment in visual perception, which is nonetheless above the level of an elementary sensory deficit such as a visual field defect. Patients do not see objects normally, and hence cannot recognize them. In contrast, associative agnosias are those in which perception seems adequate to allow recognition, and yet recognition cannot take place. It is said to involve, in the oft-quoted phrase of Teuber (1968), a "normal percept stripped of its meaning." In this respect, the apperceptive-associative distinction, as defined above, includes a significant assumption about the mechanisms of agnosia: That the underlying deficit in so-called associative agnosia lies outside of the modality-specific perceptual processing of the stimulus. Whether or not this is true is an important issue, which will be discussed later. Nevertheless, the grouping of agnosics into two categories—those with frank perceptual deficits and those without—does seem to be empirically valid. That is, the surface manifestations of agnosia in these two groups of patients differ considerably, and on that purely empirical basis they should be discussed separately.

Chapter 2
The Apperceptive Agnosias

The term apperceptive agnosia has been used to mean any failure of object recognition in which perceptual impairments seem clearly at fault, despite relatively preserved elementary visual functions such as acuity, brightness discrimination, and color vision. It has been applied to an extremely heterogeneous set of patients, whose impairments range from disorders of attention to an inability to recognize objects presented at unusual orientations. The obvious differences between these different types of patients, at the surface, behavioral level of what they can and cannot do, makes it unlikely that any theoretically useful generalizations will be drawn about this category. Therefore, some subdivision is needed.

Four types of patients will be described in this chapter, all of whom have been called apperceptive agnosics. In the case of the first three types to be discussed, the distinctions among them have not been clearly drawn in the literature. Many authors have discussed cases from more than one of these categories interchangeably (e.g., Adler, 1944; Alexander and Albert, 1983; Bauer and Rubens, 1985; Benson and Greenberg, 1969; Kertesz, 1979; Luria, 1973; Kosslyn, Flynn, Amsterdam and Wang, 1990; Williams, 1970). There are indeed certain similarities among these patients, although there are also some fundamental differences that implicate different underlying impairments in the three cases. In the case of the fourth category to be described, the use of the term apperceptive agnosia represents an intentional reappropriation of a label, used differently by other authors: Warrington (e.g., 1985) argues that most patients who have been classified as apperceptive agnosics would be better labelled "pseudoagnosics," because their perception is so extremely impaired, and that a group of patients studied extensively by her (e.g., Warrington and James, 1988) should be called apperceptive agnosics.

2.1 Apperceptive Agnosia (Narrow Sense)

A narrower use of the term "apperceptive agnosia" refers to one relatively homogeneous subgroup of these patients. These include the cases

H.C. (Adler, 1944), E.S. (Alexander and Albert, 1983), Mr. S. (Efron, 1968; Benson and Greenberg, 1969), R.C. (Campion and Latto, 1985; Campion, 1987), Schn. (Gelb and Goldstein, 1918; translated by Ellis, 1938), and X (Landis, Graves, Benson, and Hebben, 1982). Benson and Greenberg (1969) touch on many of the essential features of this syndrome in the following description of Mr. S., a young man who suffered accidental carbon monoxide (CO) poisoning.

> Visual acuity could not be measured with a Snellen eye chart, as he could neither identify letters of the alphabet nor describe their configuration. He was able to indicate the orientation of a letter "E," however, and could detect movement of a small object at standard distance. He could identify some familiar numbers if they were slowly drawn in small size on a screen. He could readily maintain optic fixation during fundoscopic examination, and optokinetic nystagmus was elicited bilaterally with fine, ⅛ inch marks on a tape . . . Visual fields were normal to 10 mm and 3 mm white objects, and showed only minimal inferior constriction bilaterally to 3 mm red and green objects. . . .
>
> The patient was able to distinguish small differences in the luminance (0.1 log unit) and wavelength (7–10 mu) of a test aperture subtending a visual angle of approximately 2 degrees. While he could detect these differences in luminance, wavelength, and area, and could respond to small movements of objects before him, he was unable to distinguish between two objects of the same luminance, wavelength, and area when the only difference between them was shape.
>
> Recent and remote memory, spontaneous speech, comprehension of spoken language, and repetition were intact. He could name colors, but was unable to name objects, pictures of objects, body parts, letters, numbers, or geometrical figures on visual confrontation. Yet he could readily identify and name objects from tactile, olfactory, or auditory cues. Confabulatory responses in visual identification utilized color and size cues (a safety pin was "silver and shiny like a watch or a nail clipper" and a rubber eraser was "a small ball"). He identified a photograph of a white typewritten letter on a blue background as "a beach scene," pointing to the blue background as "the ocean," the stationery as "the beach," and the small typewriter print as "people seen on the beach from an airplane."
>
> He consistently failed to identify or to match block letters; occasionally he "read" straight line numbers, but never those with curved parts. He could clumsily write only a few letters (X, L) and numbers

(1, 4, 7), but often inverted or reversed these. Although he could consistently identify Os or Xs as they were slowly drawn, or if the paper containing them was moved slowly before him, he was unable to identify the very same letters afterwards on the motionless page. He was totally unable to copy letters or simple figures, and he could neither describe nor trace the outline of common objects. . . .

He was unable to select his doctor or family members from a group until they spoke and was unable to identify family members from photographs. At one time he identified his own face in a mirror as his doctor's face. He did identify his own photograph, but only by the color of his military uniform. After closely inspecting a scantily attired magazine "cover girl," he surmised that she was a woman because "there is no hair on her arms." That this surmise was based on flesh color identification was evident when he failed to identify any body parts. For example, when asked to locate her eyes he pointed to her breasts. . . .(pp. 83–85)

In summary, the patient had seemingly adequate elementary visual functions and general cognitive ability, and yet he was dramatically impaired on the simplest forms of shape discrimination. Indeed, this patient was described as appearing blind to casual observers (Efron, 1968). Let us relate the findings in this case to the others mentioned above.

As was true for Mr. S., visual field defects do not seem responsible for the visual problems of the other patients in this category. In some cases the visual fields are roughly normal (Adler, 1944; Alexander and Albert, 1983; Benson and Greenberg, 1969). The remaining cases have sufficiently preserved islands of vision, on standard perimetric testing, that visual field defects do not seem an adequate explanation of their visual difficulties (Campion and Latto, 1985; Gelb and Goldstein, 1918; Landis et al., 1982). In all cases acuity is either normal or sufficient for recognition, and color vision is roughly normal, with the exception of Gelb and Goldstein's case, who was described as "not completely color blind" (Ellis, 1938, p. 316). Maintaining fixation of a visual target was possible for all but one of these cases (Alexander and Albert, 1983), and was reported difficult for one other (Adler, 1944). In the three cases in which depth perception was explicitly reported it was either intact (Gelb and Goldstein, 1918; Landis et al., 1982), or recovered while the patient was still agnosic (Adler, 1944). In two other cases we can infer that it was roughly intact from reports of normal reaching for visual objects (Campion, 1987; Efron, 1968). Three cases report roughly normal movement perception (Alexander & Albert, 1983; Benson and Greenberg, 1969; Landis et al., 1982), one case reports impaired movement perception (Gelb and

Goldstein, 1918), and the remaining cases do not give information about movement perception.

In striking contrast to their roughly intact visual sensory functions, apperceptive agnosics are severely impaired at recognizing, matching, copying or discriminating simple visual stimuli. These impairments are not subtle: Typical examples of patients' errors on such tasks include calling the numeral 9 "a capital A" (Adler, 1944), a circle "a lot of dots" (Campion, 1987), or being unable to discriminate "Xs" from "Os" (Benson and Greenberg, 1969). Figure 2 shows the attempts of two of these patients to copy simple forms. Figure 3 shows the stimuli used in two shape matching tasks that Mr. S. was unable to perform. In the first task, pairs of rectangles with the same total area were shown to the patient, and his task was to judge whether they had the same shape or a different shape. In the second task, he was asked to match a sample stimulus to one of four other stimuli which had the same shape.

The case reports give a few additional clues to the nature of these patients' perception of the visual world. For two of the cases it was mentioned that figures made up of dots were particularly hard to recognize (Gelb and Goldstein, 1918; Ellis, 1938, p. 320; Landis et al., 1982, p. 522). Three of the case reports mention greater difficulty with the perception of curved lines than straight ones (Benson and Greenberg, 1969, p. 83; Adler, 1944, p. 245; Gelb and Goldstein, 1918; Ellis, 1938, p. 322). In two of the reports it was mentioned that the patients did not seem to perceive objects as solid forms or even surfaces in three dimensions: Adler (1944, p. 252) says of her patient, "At first she perceived contours only. For example, during the second week she called a nickel and a round silver compact each 'a key ring.'" Goldstein and Gelb (Ellis, 1938, p. 318) state that "All drawings in perspective were utterly meaningless for this patient. A circle tilted away from him was invariably described as an ellipse."

Recognition of real objects is also impaired but is somewhat better than recognition of "simple" stimuli. This appears to be due to the wider set of available cues to the identity of real objects, particularly color. The patients' identifications of objects are typically *inferences*, made by piecing together color, size, texture, and reflectance clues. Mr. S.'s reliance on these properties is apparent from Benson and Greenberg's recounting of his attempts to recognize the safety pin and the picture of the typed letter. They also report that he "could select similar objects from a group only if there were strong color and size clues; after training he could name several familiar objects but failed to do so if their color and size qualities were altered. Thus he failed to identify a green toothbrush that was substituted for a previously named red toothbrush. He also called a red

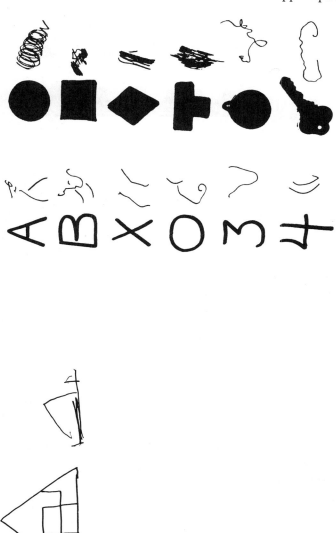

Figure 2
The copying ability of apperceptive agnosic patients. On the left is a simple geometric shape and patient E. S.'s copy. On the right are two columns of letters, numbers, and shapes, with the patient Mr. S's copies.

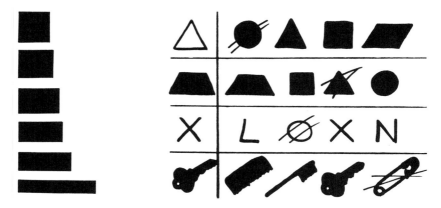

Figure 3.
The shape matching ability of apperceptive agnosic patients. On the left is a set of rectangles matched for overall area, which were presented pairwise to Mr. S. to be judged same or different in shape. He was unable to discriminate all but the most distinctive, and made errors even with these. On the right are a set of rows containing a target shape (left) and a set of four choices to be matched with the target shape. Mr. S.'s answers are marked.

pencil "my toothbrush" (p. 84). R.C. was also reported to use "features of objects such as their color or whether they were shiny or not. He could also recognize the 'texture' of objects. If encouraged, he could often make an accurate guess about the nature of objects from such cues" (Campion, 1987, p. 209). Landis et al. report similar strategies in their patient, X: "He once mentioned being on the 14th floor of the hospital. Asked how he knew, he replied "It's the only one having red exit doors." Adler's patient, too, was said to recognize objects by "a process of adding up visual impressions," and often used color to guess the identity of objects, mistaking vanilla ice cream for scrambled eggs and a piece of white soap for a piece of paper (p. 252). Even Gelb and Goldstein's patient, Schn., who had moderately impaired color vision, used color along with size to recognize objects, for example, identifying dice from their size and the presence of black dots on a white surface (Ellis, 1938, p. 324).

A striking feature of some of these cases is the spontaneous use of tracing strategies to aid in the recognition of visual stimuli. This was the most famous and controversial aspect of Gelb and Goldstein's case, who traced the contours of stimuli using both head and hand movements. With sufficient time he was able to read most print, by executing "a series of minute head and hand movements. He 'wrote' with his hand what his eyes saw. He did not move the entire hand, as if across a page, but 'wrote' the letters one over another, meanwhile 'tracing' them with head movements" (Ellis, 1938, p. 317). Gelb and Goldstein made several important observations about Schn.'s tracing behavior, which shed light on the nature of his visual abilities as well as the functional role played by tracing: "If prevented from moving his head or body, the patient could read nothing whatever . . . His movements led to reading only if they corresponded to normal writing movements. If required to trace a letter the 'wrong' way, he was quite at a loss to say what letter it was . . . If a few cross-hatching marks were drawn across the word, he followed these when he reached them and consequently lost all sense of what the word was... the scratches 'derailed' him and he was unable to rediscover the correct path . . . If the scratches were made with a different colored pencil, no difficulty was encountered; the same held for very thick letters and very thin scratches . . . It may be said that his tracing was quite 'planless', if by plan we mean guidance based on an antecedent grasp of the structure of the object to be traced. If the drawing given him to be traced were, like a circle, of such a character that he had one route to follow, the result was always successful. Not so, however, with drawings where several lines led away from a single point." (Ellis, 1938, pp. 317–318).

Critics of Gelb and Goldstein, who examined Schn. many years later, found his tracing movements rather showy and theatrical and doubted that the patient had a recognition impairment beyond such elementary visual problems as his constricted visual fields. For example, Bay (1953) and Jung (1949) noted that the patient was able to see and recognize most objects and seemed to switch into his tracing routine only when performing tests for psychologists. It is possible that the patient had recovered in the more than twenty years that had elapsed since Gelb and Goldstein's studies, and that the tracing was indeed no longer functional. The fact that other patients, with similar visual impairments, have spontaneously adopted the same type of tracing strategy makes it unlikely that the tracing was purely an affectation to attract the interest of psychologists.

Landis et al. (1982) discuss the similarity of their case X to Gelb and Goldstein's Schn. in the spontaneous use of tracing strategies. They reported that "When allowed to trace, X could recognize simple geometric figures if the point of departure for tracing was unimportant (e.g., circle, triangle). With more complex figures he was misled by unimportant lines. He would give different answers for the same drawing, dependent upon the point of starting to trace, and often described incidental background features as meaningful . . . Reading aloud was performed slowly but accurately. This "reading" was accomplished by rapid tracing of letters, parts of letters or words with his left hand alone or with both hands . . . [When] movement of the fingers could be prevented . . . this abolished reading." Also, like Gelb and Goldstein's case, X was "derailed" by slash lines, following them off of the figure being traced. Landis et al. provide another demonstration of what they call the "slavish" dependence on local continuity in their patient's tracing: When shown the stimulus in figure 4, the patient consistently read it as "7415."

Adler (1944) reports that "during the second week of her illness, the patient started to use her index finger to trace the contour of objects" (p. 244) and that even after considerable recovery, she would often "trace the contours of letters with her index finger in order to enforce perception" (p. 256). Mr. S. also spontaneously adopted a tracing strategy in a task in which he had to judge whether the orientation of two lines was the same or different. According to Efron (1968), "He carefully followed the contours of each by moving his head. Using this method, he frequently gave correct answers. However, when prevented from making head movements he could no longer perform the task" (p. 159). When asked to trace around a shape, Mr. S. "will often go round a simple figure many times, not knowing that he has completed the task . . . In those cases in which he is asked to trace a complex object, he will almost always follow the contour of a single color area" (pp 156–157). Finally, two of the cases were reported to have difficulty tracing figures by hand: Case E.S. (Alexander and Albert, 1983) had a general impairment in visually guided movements that precluded tracing, and R.C. (Campion, 1987) was reported to have difficulty tracing figures with hand movements. The latter case often resorted to spontaneous head movements when asked to identify an object, although it should be noted that Campion's interpretation was that R.C. seemed to be searching for the best view with these head movements.

Motion of the object to be recognized appears to be helpful to some of these patients. Not surprisingly, it was helpful only to those subjects who had large visual fields, as a moving object would quickly pass out of view for patients with very narrow visual fields. E.S. recognized objects best when they were "alone and moving (e.g. identifying birds or planes flying at a great distance . . .)" (Alexander and Albert, 1983, p. 408). Motion helped Mr. S. to segregate objects from their surround: "Mr. S. can point with his finger to an object which is held before him. He can do this efficiently only if the object is moved before his eyes. If it is stationary

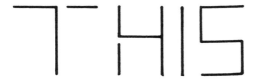

Figure 4
Patient X, studied by Landis et al. (1982), consistently read this stimulus as 7415.

he does not appear to know what object he has been asked to look at; his eyes randomly scan the entire room and he appears to be 'searching'" (Efron, 1968, p. 156). Motion also aided Mr. S.'s perception of form. Efron reports that "When I outlined a circular figure repeatedly with a pencil he was apparently able to see the shape. For a brief instant his face lit up with pleasure and he claimed that he saw the circle. A few minutes later, under static conditions, he was unable to identify the same object" (p. 159). Benson and Greenberg found that this patient was better able to recognize shapes that were moved slowly in front of him, and also that he could recognize shapes while they were being drawn, either with ink on paper (p. 83), or with a point of light on a screen (p. 85). Adler did not formally test the role of motion in H.C.'s recognition abilities, but remarked that, at the movies, "the accompanying voices and her observation of movements contribute to her understanding" (p. 253). Landis et al. (1982) tested X's recognition of written material moved in front of the patient and reported that it did not help. However, this patient normally recognized letters and words with the help of a tracing strategy, which would be foiled by stimulus movement. Therefore, the appropriate comparison would have been between moving and stationary stimuli when tracing strategies were prevented. However, like Mr. S., this patient "recognized words traced letter by letter in the air in front of him and did this much faster than any observers" (p. 522).

The neuropathology in these cases of apperceptive agnosia shows a fair degree of homogeneity. Four patients suffered carbon monoxide poisoning (Adler, 1944; Alexander and Albert, 1983; Benson and Greenberg, 1969; Campion and Latto, 1985), one suffered mercury poisoning (Landis et al., 1982), and one suffered a penetrating head wound (Gelb and Goldstein, 1918). Neurological signs, EEG, and CT scan evidence suggest that the brain damage in all of these patients was primarily posterior, affecting the occipital lobes and surrounding regions. With the exception of the penetrating head wound, the brain damage was of a diffuse and widespread rather than focal nature, and Bay (1953) suggested that the patient of Gelb and Goldstein was suffering less from the focal effects of his head wound than from increased intracranial pressure, which would also have diffuse and widespread effects. Benson and Greenberg point out that CO poisoning is known to create both diffuse cortical damage, particularly affecting the interlaminar connections between neurons, as well as multifocal disseminated lesions. Landis et al. cite research showing that mercury poisoning affects the white matter of the occipital lobe, again compromising connections between neurons to a greater degree than the neurons themselves.

To sum up the abilities and impairments of these patients, there is relative preservation of most "elementary" dimensions of visual perception, with a striking impairment in the ability to recognize, copy, or match simple shapes as well as more complex objects. Most of these patients are able to trace the shapes that they cannot recognize by vision alone, using either hand or head movements, and three of these patients spontaneously adopted tracing as a major compensatory strategy. However, the tracing has a "slavish" quality to it and consequently is useless when figures have irrelevant lines drawn through them or discontinuities in them. There is a suggestion that at least some of these patients can use information gleaned from the motion of stimuli to extract form information. The neuropathology is generally diffuse and posterior.

Many authors classify the patients just described with another group of patients who have a disorder known as "simultanagnosia" (e.g., Adler, 1944; Alexander and Albert, 1983; Bauer and Rubens, 1985; Luria, 1973). The distinction has been further muddied by the fact that simultanagnosia itself does not appear to be a homogeneous category. There are two different syndromes that have both been labelled "simultanagnosia" and discussed interchangeably, both of which are distinct from each other and from the syndrome of apperceptive agnosia reviewed above.

2.2 Dorsal Simultanagnosia

Patients with this form of simultanagnosia resemble apperceptive agnosics in that they often have full visual fields, but act as if they are blind. Furthermore, when presented with an array of stimuli, they often cannot indicate a named stimulus or identify stimuli indicated by an examiner. A final, qualitative similarity to apperceptive agnosics is that their perception has a "piecemeal" character to it: They may recognize some part or aspect of an object and guess the object's identity on the basis of the perceived feature.

The term "simultanagnosia" was originally coined by Wolpert (1924) to describe a condition in which the patient accurately perceives the individual elements or details of a complex picture, but cannot appreciate the overall meaning of the picture. Luria (1959, 1963) associated this rather general term with a specific type of perceptual deficit, in which only one object, or part of an object, can be seen at one time. This perceptual deficit is generally observed in the context of 'Balint's syndrome', which consists of (1) 'psychic paralysis of gaze', i.e., an inability to direct voluntary eye movements to visual targets, (2) optic ataxia, i.e., an inability to reach for or point to visual targets, and (3) a visual-attentional deficit in which only one stimulus at a time is perceived and even the attended stimulus may spontaneously slip from attention. The

elements of the syndrome occasionally occur separately from one another (Damasio, 1985), raising the possibility that they have different
underlying mechanisms, which are associated because of neuroanatomical proximity. It is the third element, termed simultanagnosia by Luria,
that will be discussed here. In order to distinguish this type of simultanagnosia from another syndrome that has also been called simultanagnosia, without making premature commitments to hypotheses about the
underlying mechanisms of the two disorders, I will refer to them by
associated lesion site: The disorder being discussed in this section
generally occurs after bilateral parieto-occipital damage, and so it can be
called 'dorsal simultanagnosia'. The other form of simultanagnosia is
found following left inferior occipito-temporal damage and can thus be
called 'ventral simultanagnosia'.

There are several cases of dorsal simultanagnosia in the literature that
show highly similar patterns of abilities and deficits, including the cases
of Girotti, Milanese, Casazza, Allegranza, Corridori and Avanzini (1982);
Godwin-Austen (1965); Hecaen and Ajuriaguerra (1954); Holmes (1918);
Holmes and Horrax (1919); Kase, Troncoso, Court, Tapia, and Mohr
(1977); Luria (1959); Luria, Pravdina-Vinarskaya, and Yarbuss (1963);
Tyler (1968), and Williams (1970). William's case illustrates many of the
prime features of the syndrome:

> A sixty-eight-year-old patient studied by the author had difficulty
> finding his way around because "he couldn't see properly." It was
> found that if two objects (e.g., pencils) were held in front of him at
> the same time, he could see only one of them, whether they were
> held side by side, one above the other, or one behind the other.
> Further testing showed that single stimuli representing objects or
> faces could be identified correctly and even recognized when shown
> again, whether simple or complex . . . If stimuli included more than
> one object, one only would be identified at one time, though the
> other would sometimes "come into focus" as the first one went
> out . . . If long sentences were presented, only the rightmost word
> could be read . . . If a single word covered as large a visual area as
> a sentence which could not be read, the single word was read in its
> entirety . . . If the patient was shown a page of drawings, the contents
> of which overlapped (i.e., objects were drawn on top of one an-
> other), he tended to pick out one and deny that he could see any
> others (pp. 61–62).

One of the most striking features of this syndrome is that, although
these patients are able to recognize most objects, they generally cannot
see more than one at a time. This is manifest in several ways: As with

Williams's case, many cases can name only one of a set of objects (Girotti et al., 1982; Godwin-Austen, 1965; Luria, 1959; Luria et al., 1963; Tyler, 1968). Counting is another task that requires seeing more than one object at time, in order that the subject keep track of which objects he has already counted and which he has yet to count (Godwin-Austen, 1965; Holmes, 1918; Holmes and Horrax, 1919; Luria, 1959). By contrasting visual counting ability with tactile or auditory counting ability, one can deduce whether or not the visual component of the task per se is the source of the patient's difficulty. Holmes (1918) describes the behavior of a typical case: "When asked to count a row of coins he became hopelessly confused, went from one end to the other and back again, and often passed over some of the series; but he succeeded in enumerating them correctly when he was allowed to run his left fingers over them" (p. 461). The description of complex scenes is slow and fragmentary. For example, looking out a window, Luria et al.'s (1963) patient was able to see one car at a time, saying, "I know there are many but I see only one" (p. 222). Godwin-Austen (1965) showed his patient the "telegraph boy" picture from the Binet scale, shown in figure 5, and asked her to describe it. He relates that she "first pointed out the cap, then saw and described the

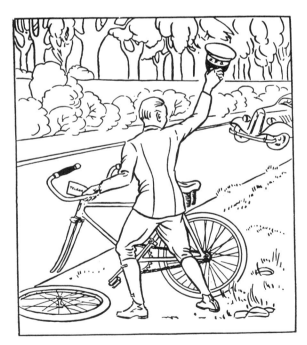

Figure 5.
The telegraph boy picture, used to assess simultanagnosia.

handlebars and the telegram, then noticed the car to the right of the picture, and finally appreciated that the telegraph boy was waving 'to something— presumably the car'. It took her nearly a minute to derive this amount of information from the picture. Until her attention was drawn to it, she failed to notice that the bicycle wheel had come off" (p. 455). When shown the scene shown in figure 6 for two seconds, Tyler's subject said she saw "a mountain." When shown the figure for another two seconds, she said "a man," and did not indicate having seen the camel, desert or pyramids, or realize that the man was related to what she had previously seen. When allowed over 30 seconds to look at the picture, she eventually said, "it's a man looking at the mountains." She said she never saw the "whole," but only bits of it that would "fade out" (p. 161). Similar complaints emerge in connection with reading: Patients complain that words pop out from the page and then disappear and are replaced by other bits of text, not necessarily adjacent to the previous bit, making reading difficult or impossible (Girotti et al., 1982; Godwin-Austen, 1965; Luria, 1959; Luria, et al. 1963; Hecaen and Ajuriaguerra, 1954, case 2; Holmes, 1918; Holmes and Horrax, 1919; Williams, 1970).

Despite this severe limitation on what they can see at one time, dorsal simultanagnosics may have full visual fields, in the sense that they are capable of detecting peripheral stimuli when their attention is correctly focussed. However, they often appear to have "shaft vision" on standard perimetric testing. Tyler describes this phenomenon in detail: "A number of attempts to plot her fields produced variable results ranging from full fields to a 4° field around the fixation point . . . [There was] an area of approximately 20° in which she recognized stimuli but showed fatiguing and eventual disappearance of the visual object in 10–30

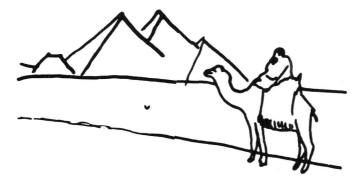

Figure 6
Drawing described by Tyler's (1968) patient as "a man looking at mountains" after prolonged scrutiny. She never noticed the camel.

seconds . . . Beyond 20° she recognized movement but any visual object faded from her awareness rapidly, and she developed a constricted field of 'effective' vision as testing persisted" (p. 158). The constriction of vision when attention is focussed is evident in situations other than perimetric field testing. For example, Hecaen and Ajuriaguerra (1954, case 1) remark that "in lighting a cigarette, when the flame was offered to him an inch or two away from the cigaratte held between his lips, he was unable to see the flame because his eyes were fixed on the cigarette" (p. 374).

These patients are often described as acting like blind people, groping for things as if in the dark, walking into furniture, and so on (Girotti et al.; Luria et al., 1963; Hecaen and Ajuriaguerra, 1954, case 1; Holmes, 1918, case 1, case 2; Kase et al., 1977). However, the impairment is clearly one of visual attention, rather than blindness or field defects, for reasons stated succinctly by Holmes and Horrax (1919): "The essential feature was his inability to . . . take cognizance of two or more objects that threw their images on the seeing part of his retinae. As this occurred no matter on what parts of his retinae the images fell, it must be attributed to a special disturbance or limitation of attention, but visual attention only was affected as he did not behave similarly to tactile or other impressions" (p. 390). Given that these patients may have full visual fields, one might wonder whether the stimuli to which these patients fail to respond are, in fact, seen at some level of awareness, perhaps just less clearly. The available evidence suggests that this is not the case. The most telling evidence is that when investigators made sudden threatening movements toward the patients' faces, the patients did not react (Godwin-Austen, 1965; Holmes, 1918, cases 1, 2, 3, 4, and 5; Holmes and Horrax, 1919). In contrast, when one of these patients' own hands was held by the experimenter and suddenly thrust toward his face, the normal reaction ensued (Holmes, 1918, case 2).

The underlying impairment in dorsal simultanagnosia appears to be a disorder of visual attention, so severe that unattended objects are not seen at all. What is the nature of this attentional limitation? Is it a limitation on the region of visual space that can be attended to, or on the number of objects that can be attended to? The answer appears to be "some of both." There is evidence that spatial extent *per se* plays some role in the attentional bottleneck. In the reports of Tyler (1968), Hecaen and Ajuriaguerra (1954), and Girotti et al. (1982) stimuli were better perceived when they subtended a small visual angle. Tyler noted that "If one put two objects in her small total field of 2° to 4° , she could recognize more than one thing at once. She could do better 'at a distance' because of this phenomenon" (p. 158). In describing a collision their patient had with a door, Hecaen and Ajuriaguerra imply that visual angle plays a role in the attentional bottleneck because the door "was too near the patient and thus did not constitute a coherent whole. The stairs [which the patient did see, at a distance of 18 yards] on the other hand, were seen in a single glance" (p. 375). Girotti et al. make a similar observation, saying that on one occasion their patient "could not clearly see people with him in the room, but he accurately identified an electrical switch placed at some meters distance from him" (p. 604). The cases of Holmes (1918) and Holmes and Horrax (1919) were able to see more than one object when the objects were contained within central vision. This points out a possible confounding between spatial compactness per se and location in the fovea in the foregoing reports. Anatomical considerations might lead us to expect different attentional mechanisms for foveal and peripheral stimuli, as the former are projected disproportionately to the inferotemporal visual pathway and the latter to the parietal pathway (e.g., Ungerleider and Mishkin, 1972). Recent work with event-related potentials recorded in normal subjects provides some more direct support for this idea: Neville and Lawson (1987) have shown that the enhancement of the visual ERP by selective attention is maximal over parietal regions of the scalp for peripheral stimuli, and occipital regions of the scalp for stimuli in central vision. In the absence of experiments with dorsal simultanagnosics contrasting foveal stimulus presentations with nonfoveal presentations subtending the same visual angle, we cannot conclude whether the limitation on visual attention in this syndrome is a limitation of size of spatial region per se or foveal spatial location per se. However, in either case the limiting factor is spatial.

An additional limitation on attention in dorsal simultanagnosia is a limitation on the number of objects that can be seen, independent of their size. Holmes and Horrax say of their patient, "It might be expected that as a result of this affection of visual attention he would be unable to see the whole of large objects presented to him at a near distance; but provided part of the image did not fall on the blind portions of his visual fields, this was never obvious on examination. He recognized objects and even complicated geometrical figures as promptly as normal persons . . . He explained this by saying 'I seem to see the whole figure in the first glance', though occasionally he failed to do so if some peculiarity or prominent portion of it at once claimed his attention" (p. 390). In the excerpt above, Williams (1970) remarks that her patient could read words no matter how large they were printed. Conversely, the patients of Tyler, Hecaen and Ajuriaguerra, and Girotti et al. failed to see small objects near another object that was the focus of their attention. Thus, beyond an occasional success with closely spaced (and probably foveal) small stimuli, these patients in general see only one object at a time, regardless of its size.

Luria and colleagues have reported a series of experiments aimed at assessing the relative contributions of number of objects and spatial extent to the attentional bottleneck in dorsal simultanagnosia. In one study (Luria et al., 1963) the patient was shown drawings of common objects at different sizes in a tachistoscope. He could name the objects presented one at a time, whether they subtended 6°–8° or 15°–20°. (Note that these sizes are much larger than the fovea.) However, when two were shown simultaneously, even at the smaller size, the patient could only name one. In another study with a different patient, Luria (1959) reports that two forms were more likely to be perceived if connected by a line drawn between them, an observation also made by Godwin-Austen (1965). Luria (1959) presented two different versions of a Star of David to his patient, asking the patient to name what he saw. In the first version, the star was drawn all in the same color of ink. In the second, one of the two component triangles was drawn in red and the other was drawn in blue. The second version provided a stimulus in which there were two distinct "objects" or visual gestalts, the red and blue triangles, occupying roughly the same region of space as each other, and together occupying precisely the same region of space as the first version of the star. When shown the first version, the patient consistently named the star. When shown the second version, the patient either named the red triangle or the blue triangle. This finding demonstrates the importance of number of objects per se, rather than sheer visual area or visual complexity (measured in number of contours) in the allocation of attention. Luria also reports that the patient could recognize a tachistoscopically presented line drawing of a face so long as the entire face was drawn in the same color ink; when different parts were drawn in different colors, he was unable to see the whole face.

To the extent that attention is allocated to objects, as opposed to locations or regions of space, this raises the question of what an object is, from the point of view of the attentional systems of dorsal simultanagnosics. The experimental findings of Luria, along with the clinical observations of several other writers described above, suggest that "objecthood" is not simply a matter of size or of visual complexity. Another demonstration that what counts as an object is not determined by simple physical stimulus properties is the following observation of Luria (1959): When his patient was shown a rectangle made up of six dots, the patient was unable to count the dots. Recall that dorsal simultanagnosics cannot count objects because this requires seeing more than one object at a time. In contrast, this patient could see the rectangle made up of the six dots, as well as recognize other geometric forms drawn with broken lines. Apparently the patient could view the stimulus as dots, and hence see a single dot at a time, or he could view it as a rectangle, and hence see the entire rectangle. In the latter case, the patient was still unable to count the dots, presumably because once he started to count the dots, he would again be seeing them as dots and see only one at a time. In other words, the organization of the dots into a rectangle did not increase the patient's attentional capacity to more than one object; rather, it allowed the patient to view the set of dots as a single object. An implication of this is that the attentional system of dorsal simultanagnosics is sensitive to voluntary, "top-down" determinants of what constitutes an object.

With real objects, as with patterns of dots, there is some flexibility possible in what we take to be an object, as opposed to a collection of objects or a part of an object. For example, a face can be viewed as an object, a collection of other objects such as eyes, nose, and mouth, or as a part of a larger object, the human body. Indeed, the patient described by Luria et al. (1963) "immediately perceived a face, [but] he was unable to concentrate his gaze on the separate details for, when a detail was perceived, its relation to the whole was immediately lost" (p. 224). Apparently, whatever attentional process is disrupted in dorsal simul-tanagnosia is sensitive to these shifts in what the visual system takes to be an "object."

Tyler observed a related phenomenon in his patient, who would some-times see only a part of a stimulus and guess at its identity based on that part. For example, "When shown a pitcher pouring water into a glass, she first noted the handle and said 'suitcase'. When asked to look again she spotted the glass, and remembering the handle she kept looking until she perceived the pitcher (now with the handle on it)" (Tyler, 1968, p. 158). This is reminiscent of Holmes and Horrax's comment that their patient sometimes failed to see a whole object if "some peculiarity or prominent portion of it at once claimed his attention." Tyler's patient's description of her visual experience, when shown a picture of the American flag, was as follows: "I see a lot of lines. Now I see some stars. When I see things like this, I see a lot of parts. It's like you have one part here and one part there, and you put them together to see what they make." Many objects have parts that can themselves be seen as objects, for example the stars or stripes on the flag, and as a result, dorsal simultanagnosics may sometimes seem to have difficulty in recognizing objects. However, it is more accurate to say that they have difficulty *seeing* objects, or seeing them at the "correct" level of the hierarchy of part-whole analysis; whatever they can see they can recognize. Furthermore, such problems are rare, as their attention is almost always claimed by a single whole object.

There are some reports that suggest that, even when dorsal simultan-agnosics succeed in seeing an object, they often "lose" it. One way this can occur is if the object is moving. Godwin-Austen (1965) reports that his patient was "unable to follow a moving object with her eyes, tending to 'lose' it and then searching with her eyes until it was located again" (p. 454). This is consistent with the report of Girotti et al. that their patient, "while watching a car race on television . . . could distinguish an advertisement on the screen but he neither saw nor identified the rapidly running racing cars" (p. 604). Although both Luria et al. and Holmes and Horrax report that slow, regular movement of an object causes no problems, Holmes and Horrax add that irregular, unpredictable move-ment causes the object to "disappear." In addition, some patients intro-spect that stationary objects seem to disappear spontaneously (Godwin-Austen, 1965; Luria, 1959; Tyler, 1968).

Recently Rizzo and Hurtig (1987) studied the eye movements and subjective visual reports of three patients with dorsal simultanagnosia who experienced the disappearance of stationary visual stimuli from direct view. They found that in all three cases, patients reported that stimuli disappeared while they were continuing to fixate them directly. Thus, the reports of stimulus disappearance in simultanagnosia is not secondary to eye movement problems. On the contrary, the tendency of these patients to make erratic, searching eye movements seems due, at least sometimes, to the spontaneous disappearance of the object they were viewing.

One last characteristic of dorsal simultanagnosia that should be noted here is the inability to localize stimuli, *even when the stimuli are seen*. This may be demonstrated by asking the subjects to point to or reach for a visual stimulus that they can see (e.g. Girotti et al., 1982; Godwin-Austen, 1965; Hecaen and Ajuriaguerra, 1954, cases 1, 2, 3, and 4; Holmes, 1989, cases 1, 2, 3, 4, and 5; Holmes and Horrax, 1919; Kase et al., 1977, cases 1 and 2; Luria, 1959; Tyler, 1968) or to describe its location relative to another object (e.g. Godwin-Austen, 1965; Holmes, 1989, cases 1, 2 and 6; Holmes and Horrax, 1919; Kase et al., case 1, case 2). The problem is not in pointing or in describing locations per se, as the patient may be able to locate auditory stimuli (Godwin-Austen, 1965; Holmes, 1918, case 3; Holmes and Horrax, 1919) or named or touched body parts (Holmes and Horrax, 1919; Kase et al., 1977, case 1) in these ways with great precision. This impairment has been termed "visual disorientation."

The brain damage that causes dorsal simultanagnosia is bilateral and generally includes the parietal and superior occipital regions. In a few cases there has been evidence of damage confined to the occipital regions (Girotti et al., 1982; Rizzo and Hurtig, 1987), although, in another, only the superior parietal lobes were damaged (Kase et al., 1977, case 1).

In summary, patients with dorsal simultanagnosia have full or nearly full visual fields but can usually see only one object at a time. Other objects, even occupying the same general region of space, are not perceived. Occasionally, more than one small object in central vision can be perceived. Moving objects may be particularly difficult to maintain perception of, but even stationary objects currently in view may spontaneously disappear. Dorsal simultanagnosics have difficulty localizing objects in space. However, so long as they can see an object, they can recognize it.

2.3 Ventral Simultanagnosia

There is another group of patients who have been called simultanagnosics, whose lesions are in the left inferior temporo-occipital region. I will refer to this form of simultanagnosia as "ventral simultanagnosia." Ventral simultanagnosia shares the following characteristics with dorsal simultanagnosia: Patients are generally able to recognize a single object, but do poorly with more than one, and with complex pictures. Their introspections sound strikingly similar to those of dorsal simultanagnosics: For example, when viewing a complex picture, one patient said "I can't see it all at once. It comes to me by casting my eye around" (Kinsbourne and Warrington, 1962, p. 466). As in dorsal simultanagnosia, reading is severely impaired. Furthermore, as in dorsal simultanagnosia, the size of the objects do not matter; the limitation is in the number of objects per se (Kinsbourne and Warrington, 1962). It is therefore not surprising that the same label has been applied to these patients. Indeed, they are often discussed interchangeably (Bauer and Rubens, 1985; Benson and Greenberg, 1969; De Renzi, 1982; Frederiks, 1969; Kertesz, 1987; Kosslyn et al., 1990; Williams, 1970). However, on closer inspection the abilities and deficits of these two groups of patients differ in important ways, implicating different underlying impairments.

Although ventral simultanagnosics cannot recognize multiple objects, they differ from dorsal simultanagnosics in that they can *see* mutiple objects. This is evident in their ability to count scattered dots (Kinsbourne and Warrington, 1962), as well as in their ability to manipulate objects and walk around without bumping into obstacles. Furthermore, given sufficient time, they can also recognize multiple objects. The most obvious manifestation of their perceptual impairment is in reading. They tend to read words slowly, a letter at a time, earning them the labels "letter-by-letter readers" or "spelling dyslexics" because they spell words before recognizing them. They also perform abnormally when asked to describe complex pictures: They respond slowly, describing individual elements of the picture, often without showing any understanding of the scene as a whole. For example, when asked to describe the drawing shown in figure 5, a patient studied by Kinsbourne and Warrington (1962) said "A bicycle with the wheel off. Cranks. Pedal. Back wheel. A young chap sitting on the bike. Something he is carrying on the bike . . ." (p. 466). There have been three detailed studies of the visual capabilties of these patients, which provide many insights into the underlying nature of the disorder. Each will be summarized here.

Kinsbourne and Warrington (1962) compared the tachistoscopic recognition thresholds for letters presented singly and in pairs for four ventral simultanagnosics. There was little difference between the thresholds of the simultanagnosics and both normal and brain-damaged control subjects for recognizing single letters. However, whereas the exposure duration needed by the control subjects to recognize two letters presented simultaneously was only slightly longer, it was an order of magnitude longer for the simultanagnosics. Kinsbourne and Warrington repeated this procedure with the simultanagnosics using geometric forms and simple drawings of objects and found the same pattern of performance: Greatly elevated thresholds when two items rather than one had to be identified. By varying the size and position of the two items, they determined that neither of these factors played a role in the perceptual limitation of their patients. That is, it is not the case that ventral simultanagnosics have trouble recognizing items in particular positions or over too broad a region of the visual field. Rather, they have trouble recognizing more than one object per se. Finally, Kinsbourne and Warrington presented pairs of forms sequentially and found that simultanagnosics were also impaired at recognizing multiple stimuli even when the stimuli were not strictly simultaneous. They independently varied the intervals between the onsets of the two stimuli, the duration of the stimulus presentations, and the duration of the blank interval between the stimuli, and found that performance depended solely on the total time available for stimulus processing, that is, the length of time between the onset of the first stimulus and the offset of the second. It should be noted that they did not follow their stimulus presentations with a mask of any sort, so that the difference between stimulus exposure time and blank interstimulus interval time cannot be assumed to affect the amount of perceptual processing of the stimulus. Kinsbourne and Warrington concluded from the results of their experiments that the underlying problem in simultanagnosia is an elevated "refractory period" between the recognition of multiple forms.

Levine and Calvanio (1978) studied three ventral simultanagnosic patients in a series of tachistoscopic recognition tasks that confirm and extend the basic observations of Kinsbourne and Warrington. The patients' tachistoscopic recognition thresholds for single letters were no longer than those of age-matched normal subjects, as would be expected from Kinsbourne and Warrington's results. Furthermore, Levine and Calvanio showed this to be true even when the letters were masked. The patients also did predictably poorly, relative to normal subjects, at reading arrays of three letters, although three-letter words were read more successfully than three-letter nonsense strings. When given a pre-cue designating which letter-position should be read (i.e., the left, middle, or right), the patients performed much better with the three-letter arrays. When the position cue came after the presentation of the three letters, their performance dropped back to the same level as when no position cue was given, implying that the cue had its effect during the perception of the stimuli. In order to better separate recognition from naming operations, Levine and Calvanio presented their patients with a matching task, in which three letters were presented and patients were to say whether the array contained two identical letters or not, without having to name the letters. The patients were impaired in this task, too, implying that the deficit is in visual recognition of multiple forms. This conclusion is also supported by the effects of visual similarity among the letters on performance on this task. If the triad on a matching trial consisted of visually similar letters, e.g., "OCO," patients performed worse than if the triad consisted of visually dissimilar letters, e.g., "OXO," implying that the locus of impaired processing was visual. Similarly, more recent data briefly described by Levine and Calvanio (1982) show that the visual complexity of letters is also a determinant of ventral simultanagnosics' errors: More errors are made on strings such as "RWK" than "DVT."

Warrington and Rabin (1971) conducted a large group study of focally brain-damaged patients on the same type of task used by Kinsbourne and Warrington: The recognition of multiple, briefly displayed characters. By testing patients selected for lesion site, rather than simultanagnosia, they intended to test the localization inferred by Kinsbourne and Warrington on the basis of clinical findings in two cases (Kinsbourne and Warrington, 1962) and autopsy findings in one case (Kinsbourne and Warrington, 1963). By comparing performance on "nonverbal" stimuli (lines of different orientations and curvatures) as well as on numbers and letters, they intended to verify that the impairment extends to nonverbal as well as verbal materials. Finally, by manipulating the similarity of the letter strings to English, they intended to discriminate between two possible loci for the impairment: perception, and short-term memory. The experimenters reasoned that if the similarity of the letter sequences to familiar sequences has an effect on the degree of impairment, then the impairment must lie in memory systems, where knowledge is known to affect processing, rather than in perception. The letter strings used in this research were random, second-, and fourth-order statistical approximations to English, which show increasing similarity to the sequences of letters that make up English words.

Warrington and Rabin found that the left posterior patients were the most impaired at the span tasks, including the nonverbal one, supporting earlier conclusions about the localization of simultanagnosia and its generality beyond alphanumeric stimuli. In addition, they found effects of familiarity on the performance of all patients, including the impaired left posterior group, and from this concluded that the left posterior-damaged patients had an impairment in visual short-term memory. This finding is consistent with Levine and Calvanio's (1978) later finding that simultanagnosic patients can read more letters when the letters make words than when they make nonwords. Unfortunately, the interpretation of such results is less straightforward than might at first appear. One difficulty is that one might as easily argue that finding a normal effect of familiarity implies that the impairment must *not* be in short-term memory as to argue that short-term memory is implicated as the locus of impairment. That is, if a variable that is believed to affect a particular processing stage has just as much of an effect when task performance is impaired as when it is normal, one could argue that the impaired performance is not due to changes in that particular processing stage: The normal effect of the variable in question could be taken as evidence of normal processing at that stage. Whether one should expect to find normal effects of a variable like familiarity in patients with short-term memory impairments, or greater or smaller effects, depends upon the model one has of the role of familiarity in short-term memory, the role of short-term memory in performance of the task, and the nature of the hypothesized short-term memory impairment. These kinds of conditions are rarely met in neuropsychology research, for an assortment of reasons, not the least of which is that the relevant cognitive psychology models do not exist in many cases. A second difficulty with Warrington and Rabin's conclusion that a short-term memory impairment underlies simultanagnosia is that familiarity effects need not be limited to post-perceptual processing. In chapter 3 we will consider in more detail the ways in which "top-down" effects of familiarity can affect visual perception.

2.4 Apperceptive Agnosia, Dorsal and Ventral Simultanagnosia: Similarities and Differences

I have argued that there are three distinct syndromes whose boundaries should be taken seriously for purposes of neuropsychological theorizing, but which are often discussed interchangeably in just such contexts. Given the "family resemblance" among these syndromes, it is not hard to understand why their boundaries have often been ignored. Apperceptive agnosics and dorsal simultanagnosics share many characteristics: They may act effectively blind, being unable to negotiate visual environments of any complexity, colliding with obstacles, making random searching eye movements if asked to look at a particular object, etc., even though they may have normal visual fields, acuity, and color perception. Their perception appears to be piecemeal and confined to a local part or region of the visual field. Although apperceptive agnosics may seem generally more impaired at recognizing objects, both types of patients may evince object recognition difficulties and, when encountering these difficulties, both typically resort to guessing based on correct partial perceptions. The neuropathology does not provide a clear basis for distinguishing among these patients. In both groups it is bilateral, posterior, and spares striate cortex to at least some degree, with cases of focal parieto-occipital damage occurring in both groups.

Similarly, ventral simultanagnosics share characteristics with these patients: They, too, perceive complex visual stimuli in a piecemeal manner, and a reading impairment is prominent in all three types of patients. Like dorsal simultanagnosics, the limitation on what they perceive is not determined by size or position but by number of objects. Although the neuropathology of ventral simultanagnosia appears quite different from that of dorsal simultanagnosia, apparently this discrepancy at the neuropathological level has impressed researchers less than the similarity at the behavioral level. For example, Bauer and Rubens (1985, pp. 193–194) discuss Levine and Calvanio's (1978) results as being relevant to the simultanagnosia found in Balint's syndrome, citing the cases of Luria (1959) and Hecaen and Ajuriaguerra (1954) as examples. They also refer to Kinsbourne and Warrington's (1962) cases as having "a mild form" of the defect present in the two dorsal cases just mentioned. Many other researchers have discussed cases with these two disorders interchangeably (Benson and Greenberg, 1969; De Renzi, 1982; Frederiks, 1969; Kertesz, 1987; Kosslyn et al., in press; Williams, 1970).

Despite these similarities, a closer look at the abilities and impairments of these groups of patients leads to the conclusion that the underlying deficits must be very different. Consider the "piecemeal" nature of perception in each case. In apperceptive agnosia only very local contour is perceived. It is so local that patients cannot trace across a break in a line, trace dotted lines, or avoid "derailment" onto irrelevant slashes drawn across a figure. This is not at all the case in dorsal simultanagnosia. Whole shapes are perceived, even if composed of dots or broken lines. What is piecemeal about the perception of dorsal simultanagnosics is the limitation of their vision to a single object or visual gestalt, without awareness of the presence or absence of other stimuli. Furthermore, in dorsal simultanagnosia the nature of the "piece" is at least partially determined by conscious attention (e.g., to the individual dots arranged in a rectangle or to the rectangle), whereas no such top-down influences have been noted to affect the piecemeal perception of apperceptive agnosics. In ventral simultanagnosia, *recognition* is piecemeal, that is, limited to one object at a time, although in contrast to dorsal simultanagnosia, other objects are *seen*. The guessing strategies of apperceptive agnosics and dorsal simultanagnosics are likewise similar only on the surface. Although both make educated guesses about objects' identities based on partial perceptual information, the nature of the information used by each is different. Apperceptive agnosics use color, size, and texture, but do not use shape information. Dorsal simultanagnosics do use shape information. Furthermore, the shape perception of dorsal simultanagnosics is intact. A final difference is that, whereas motion tends to facilitate shape perception by apperceptive agnosics, it interferes with perception by dorsal simultanagnosics.

2.5 Perceptual Categorization Deficit

The patients in the foregoing three categories of apperceptive agnosia have clinically evident problems with vision, and most of what is known about them comes from clinical case descriptions. A fourth use of the term "apperceptive agnosia" refers to patients whose visual problems must be elicited experimentally. This form of apperceptive agnosia has often been studied in groups of patients delineated by lesion site as well as in individual cases selected for their poor performance on the relevant tests.

The most salient feature of these patients, first noted by De Renzi, Scotti and Spinnler (1969), is that they have great difficulty matching three-dimensional objects across shifts of perspective. In De Renzi et al.'s study, the objects being matched were faces, and the poorest performance on this task was found in right hemisphere-damaged patients with visual field defects, implying that the critical lesions were in the posterior right hemisphere. Warrington and her colleagues have demonstrated that this impairment extends to objects other than faces, and to the task of simply naming a common object viewed from an unusual perspective as well as matching across perspective shifts. For example, Warrington and Taylor (1973) showed that right posteriorly damaged patients were no worse than normal subjects at naming objects photographed from conventional views like that shown in figure 7a, but were, on average, quite poor at naming the same objects photographed from unconventional views like that shown in figure 7b. Warrington and Taylor (1978) found that even when patients had recognized the conventional view,

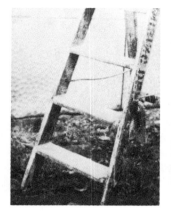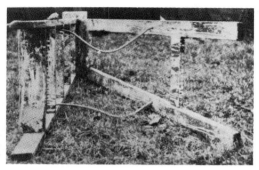

Figure 7
Usual and unusual views.

they were sometimes unable to see that the corresponding unconventional view was the same object in a matching task. Warrington and James (1986) found that the kind of perspective change did not affect these patients' ease of recognition. They presented silhouettes created by back-illuminating objects and gradually rotated the objects from an unconventional perspective to the conventional one. They found that the axis of rotation did not matter: patients were no more impaired when the unconventional perspective caused extreme foreshortening along the axis of elongation than when it preserved the axis of elongation. Under both kinds of transformations, the patients required greater rotation toward the conventional perspective before recognizing the object from its silhouette than did the normal subjects. The critical lesion site for this impairment, based on superimposed reconstructions of lesions in Warrington and Taylor's (1973) study, appears to be the right posterior inferior parietal lobe.

Although most attention has been paid to the effects of differing perspectives on the ability of these patients to recognize and match photographed objects, Warrington (1985) points out that other manipulations of perceptual quality also pose problems for these patients. She cites unpublished data of Warrington and Ackroyd demonstrating that the matching impairment extends to photographs of objects with uneven lighting, for example, the pair of pictures shown in figure 8. Warrington therefore describes the impairment in a fairly general way, as a failure of "perceptual categorization," rather than a failure of orientation invariance, suggesting that patients can no longer categorize perceptually dissimilar images in terms of the distal stimulus object that they have in common.

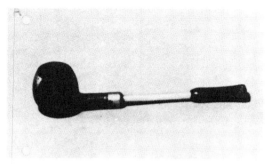

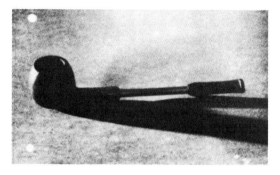

Figure 8
Evenly and unevenly lit views.

In addition to the group studies just described, in which a large number of brain-damaged patients are grouped by hemisphere or quadrant of damage, and some summary measure of the performance of these anatomically defined groups is compared with the performance of control subjects, there have also been case studies of perceptual categorization deficit. Warrington and James (1988) present three cases of what they term "apperceptive agnosia": Right posteriorly damaged patients who performed within normal limits on tests of elementary visual function, including the Efron (1968) rectangle matching task (see p. 12), but performed extremely poorly on a series of tests of perceptual categorization. They were able to recognize only 6–8 out of 20 unconventional views of objects, like the photograph in figure 7b, although they named almost all of the same objects (17–20 out of 20) when shown them later from conventional perspectives, like the photograph in figure 7a. When asked to name silhouettes of objects in an unconventional foreshortened orientation, and when shown the silhouettes of objects being rotated from unconventional to conventional perspectives, they made many errors and required that the object be rotated to a more conventional perspective before being able to identify it.

In an effort to distinguish between two distinct processes that might underlie perceptual categorization, Humphreys and Riddoch (1984, 1985) manipulated the recognizability of objects seen from unconventional views in two ways: by foreshortening the major axes of elongation, and by reducing the number or salience of characteristic features of the object. Whereas the four right-hemisphere-damaged patients they tested had more difficulty recognizing the foreshortened views than the minimal feature views, a bilaterally damaged associative agnosic patient (H.J.A., who will be discussed in chapter 4) showed the opposite trend in his performance. This suggests that there may be two different processes by which visual stimuli are perceptually categorized, one relying primarily on the overall geometry of the image and one on the features visible in the image. This interpretation, as well as other hypotheses about the processes underlying perceptual categorization, will be discussed in the next chapter.

In summary, damage to the right posterior quadrant of the brain, especially the right posterior inferior parietal lobe, is associated with difficulty in perceiving the intrinsic shape of an object when the perspective is unconventional or the lighting uneven. This has been termed "apperceptive agnosia" by Warrington and her colleagues, as well as a "perceptual categorization" deficit.

Chapter 3

Interpreting the Apperceptive Agnosias in Terms of Theories of Normal Visual Object Recognition

3.1 Apperceptive Agnosia (Narrow Sense)

Apperceptive agnosics are impaired at just about all visual abilities involving the perception of shape: They cannot match shapes, recognize them, name them, or shift their attention to a named shape to verify that it is present, even though they can perceive local contour fairly accurately. Several writers have speculated about how the abilities and deficits of these patients can be explained in terms of theories of normal object recognition. For example, Benson and Greenberg (1969) note the similarity of their case to Adler's (1944) case, and propose that both involved a specific loss of form perception. Although this seems correct, it does not go very far beyond a redescription of the data themselves.

3.1.1 The masking hypothesis

Campion and Latto (1985) attempt to give a more explanatory account of the deficits shown by their case, as well Adler's and Benson and Greenberg's. They point out that their patient's visual field was "peppered" by small scotomata, as shown in figure 9, and that this might well be the case with the other two patients, too, given the tendency of carbon monoxide (CO) to produce many small, disseminated lesions. According to Campion and Latto, form perception would be impaired by viewing stimuli through a peppery "mask." Humphreys and Riddoch (1987b) endorse this view in their taxonomy of agnosia, calling the three patients discussed by Campion and Latto "shape agnosics" and saying that the underlying deficit in these cases is that the "initial registration of the elements of form perception seems impaired . . . there may be many small areas of decreased sensitivity or even blindness in the patients' visual fields, impairing the registration of forms which fall across these areas" (p. 105). A prediction of this hypothesis is that normal subjects would behave like apperceptive agnosics when viewing the world through a peppery mask. Campion and Latto demonstrate that such masking does interfere with normal subjects' ability to identify photographed objects

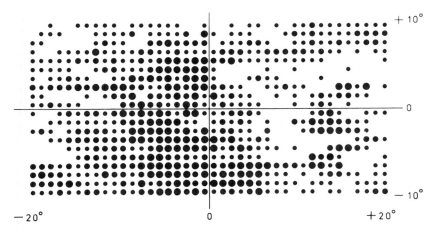

Figure 9
Representation of patient R.C.'s visual field, in which dot size represents the rated brightness of light targets. A large spot indicates low rated brightness.

and scenes, and offer the pair of pictures shown in figure 10 as a means for the reader to verify this personally.

This explanation is elegant in its simplicity and in its correspondence with the neuropathological findings in these cases. However, on closer examination, it leaves several questions unanswered. First, it is not clear how the masking hypothesis accounts for the quality of the apperceptive agnosic's difficulties, specifically the extreme *locality* of perception in these cases. That is, whereas the visual recognition ability of normal subjects is impaired by superposition of a peppery mask, it has not been demonstrated that it is impaired in a way similar to the perception of apperceptive agnosics. Although grey-scale photographs are rendered quite difficult to recognize by a peppery mask, why would the perception of simple, high-contrast geometric forms, such as the rectangles shown in figure 3, be so profoundly disrupted? Why would a peppery mask interfere disproportionately with the ability to perceive a form with a slash through it (compared to the same form without a slash), or to trace past a break in a line? The deletion of many random bits of a geometric figure would seem to encourage greater reliance on global shape properties such as "good continuity," rather than inducing a slavish reliance on local bits of contour. Second, although figure 9 does indeed look "peppery," examination of the scale reveals that the scotomata are large and, more relevant, the islands of preserved vision within the central 40° by 20° are large enough to accomodate at least some single objects or designs on paper quite comfortably. Thus, at least for case R.C., the

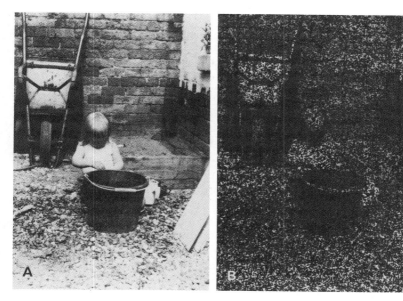

Figure 10
A photograph of a scene with and without a "peppery" mask. The mask is intended to simulate the visual impairment of apperceptive agnosics according to Campion and Latto's (1985) theory.

masking hypothesis would seem to predict good perception of stimuli in particular locations. Perhaps some more refined version of the masking hypothesis could deal with these issues; at present, however, it does not seem to be a complete explanation of apperceptive agnosia.

3.1.2 Grouping processes

Although the underlying impairment in apperceptive agnosia need not be in shape representation per se, it must be in some process that is required for shape representation. The inability of these patients to trace past a small break in a line or to trace dotted lines suggests that the impairment may have a functional locus considerably earlier than shape recognition. One thing that shape recognition as well as the seemingly easy task of tracing have in common is the necessity for *grouping* together the separately registered elements of contour into higher order units, either larger scale contours, regions, or surfaces. Normal subjects are quite adept at extracting form under conditions of partial occlusion, either by slashes or gaps in a figure or by a peppery mask. Our ability to do this has generally been attributed to "grouping processes." The gestaltists believed that grouping together elements of the visual field, on the basis of such perceptual properties as proximity, similarity, and good continuity was a fundamental stage in visual perception. In Marr's (1982) theory, grouping processes operate on the raw primal sketch to form the first step out of the extreme locality of early vision, yielding representations of the larger scale structure of the visual field. The shifting, scintillating structure apparent in figure 11 is the result of rivalrous grouping processes actively organizing the local elements of the figure. Figure 12 illustrates some of the ways grouping processes lead to higher order shape tokens in the "full primal sketch" in Marr's theory: In each diagram, a group of local form elements is being combined and treated as a single unit. The underlying impairment in apperceptive agnosics appears to lie in their grouping processes, in that they have adequate perception of local properties of the visual field (color, brightness, depth, and contour elements), but generally cannot perceive higher order shape tokens. Their limited ability to do so is extremely fragile, being disrupted by the addition of slashes or breaks in lines, and is often mediated by kinesthetic cues. Like the masking account, this account is also consistent with the neuropathology. The implication of relatively more white matter than grey matter damage in several of these cases accords well with the view that grouping processes, which would depend upon interactions between neighboring neurons, are impaired. Of course, this

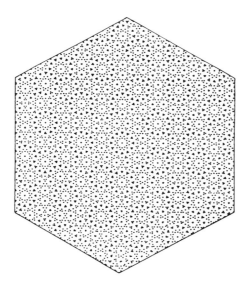

Figure 11
A demonstration of grouping processes at work. The shifting, seething patterns seen here are the result of rivalrous grouping processes.

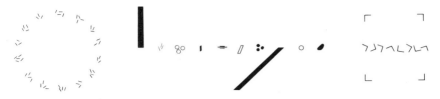

Figure 12
Examples of a few ways in which local elements of the visual field can be grouped into higher-order shape tokens.

account needs to be made more precise and tested with new evidence. Ideally, the predictions of specific grouping algorithms for the relative difficulty of perceiving different kinds of stimuli (curved versus straight lines, broken lines with different amounts of contour missing, etc.) could be compared with patients' ability to recognize these stimuli.

3.1.3 Independence of form from motion

Another characteristic of apperceptive agnosics that relates to current theories of vision is their relatively preserved use of visual motion for perception of form. This is counterintuitive if one believes that "form perception is form perception," but is consistent with recent findings implicating separate channels for the perception of form from static contour and from motion. Whereas the perception of static form is dependent on visual areas in the ventral visual pathway, going from the occipital lobe into the inferior temporal lobe, recent work on the posterior parietal lobe, in the dorsal visual pathway, has shown this area to be important for the perception of structure from motion (Andersen, 1989). The suggestion in some of these case reports of preserved ability to perceive the shapes of moving objects, and to perceive shapes traced out in motion implies that there is some independence between the grouping of local visual elements based on purely *spatial* factors such as proximity, and *spatiotemporal* factors involved in perceiving the correlated nature of rigid body motion or the shape of a path traced in time. It does not necessarily imply that motion-based grouping occurs prior to spatially based grouping; in fact the neurophysiology of motion perception implies that it occurs later. The present data imply only that grouping based on motion need not depend upon the results of grouping based on spatial structure. If the lateral interactions needed for spatially based grouping in the occipital lobe were compromised, but the local form information were being passed on to the parietal motion perception areas, this is what one would expect.

3.2 Dorsal Simultanagnosia

3.2.1 Characterizing the attentional functions of the dorsal visual system

The patients classified here as dorsal simultanagnosics have generally been described in their case reports as suffering from a limitation of visual attention. What exactly is meant by "visual attention" in this context? And, what can we learn about visual attention from the behavior of dorsal simultanagnosics?

Luria had one specific meaning of the term visual attention in mind in his research on dorsal simultanagnosia. He suggested that the attentional deficit in these patients consists of diminished "excitability" of visual cortex, so that the cortex can respond to, at most, one stimulus at a time. Luria tested this hypothesis by administering caffeine to one dorsal simultanagnosic patient (Luria, 1959) and galentamine to another (Luria et al., 1963), on the assumption that these drugs would increase neuronal excitability. The patients' perception reportedly did improve under the influence of these drugs. The results of this experiment are difficult to interpret, however, without a better understanding of some of the assumptions of Luria's hypothesis: It is not clear just what neuronal "excitability" means, in physiological or in information-processing terms, or why a limitation in excitability would be manifest in the number of objects that can be seen at one time, rather than in the clarity or vividness of perception or the size of the region of visual field that can be seen at one time. It should be added that Tyler (1968) was unable to replicate Luria's drug effects with his own subject.

Recent work by Posner and his associates suggests another, more specific interpretation of dorsal simultanagnosia in terms of a disorder of visual attention. In early research by this group (e.g., Posner, Friedrich, Walker, and Rafal, 1984), unilaterally parietal-damaged patients were given a simple reaction time task, in which a "target" stimulus would appear in one of two positions, to the left or right of a fixation point, and the subject was to press a button as soon as a target appeared. On some trials, the target was preceded by a "cue" stimulus in one of the two possible target locations. Subjects were told not to respond to the cue, and in some conditions the cue was not even predictive of the location of the upcoming target. Nevertheless, both brain-damaged and normal subjects show an effect of the cue, with responses to the target being faster when the cue and target are on the same side, indicating that the cue stimulus automatically attracts attention to itself, whether or not it is predictive of the target location. Parietal-damaged subjects differed from control subjects primarily in one condition: When the cue appeared on the side of space ipsilateral to the lesion, and the target then appeared on the side of space contralateral to the lesion, response times to the target were greatly elevated. Posner et al. interpret this finding in terms of the role of the parietal lobe in *disengaging* attention. That is, for a new stimulus to be able to engage attention, the contralateral parietal lobe must first disengage attention from its current location. More recent research has shown that the problem of unilaterally parietal-damaged patients is not limited to disengaging attention from stimuli in the ipsilateral hemifield; these patients are impaired at disengaging attention from any location (ipsilateral or contralateral) in order to reengage it at a new location in the contralateral hemifield (Baynes, Holtzman and Volpe, 1986). If we extrapolate this finding to the case of bilateral parietal damage, we would predict that once attention had been engaged by a stimulus, no other stimulus in either hemifield would be able to attract attention to itself. This describes the basic phenomena of dorsal simultanagnosia, namely, the inability to see more than one thing at a time, and the inability to shift attention from one stimulus to another. Note that this account does not postulate *diminished* visual attention, but rather abnormally "sticky" visual attention. Of course, this interpretation needs to be tested directly with dorsal simultanagnosics in a cued simple reaction time task.

The hypothesis that dorsal simultanagnosia consists of a bilateral disengage deficit also helps explain why stimuli that have been successfully fixated by these patients are wont to disappear, as reported in several case studies and carefully verified in the study of Rizzo and Hurtig (1987). Prolonged and uninterrupted fixation by normal subjects will result in the subjective disappearance of stimuli (the Troxler effect, see Kaufman, 1974, chapter 10), presumably through adaptation of representations in the visual system. The inability of dorsal simultanagnosics to disengage attention from a stimulus would result in just the conditions that give rise to the Troxler effect in normal subjects.

3.2.2 Attention to objects and locations

What about the finding that the visual attention of dorsal simultanagnosics is primarily limited to a single object, with some, relatively weaker, limitation on spatial extent? Most discussions of visual neglect, as well as those of visual attention more generally, include the assumption that attention is allocated to locations in space, rather than to objects. However, given the natural confounding between objects and their locations in most experiments, most of the data currently at hand do not distinguish between these alternatives. Neisser (1967) proposed an alternative view, according to which preattentive grouping processes formed objects from the field of local contour, color, and other attributes, which focal attention could then select, one object at a time, for further processing. Duncan (1984) reports a series of experiments in which the predictions of the hypotheses that attention is allocated to locations and to objects are contrasted, and found evidence favoring object-based attention: When two objects occupy roughly the same location, subjects can report two different attributes of one object as easily as one, but cannot report two attributes that come from different objects without a drop in performance. This is predicted by the object-based attention hypothesis but not by the location-based hypothesis because the distances between the pairs of same-object and different-object attributes were the same. Duncan notes that his results do not rule out the possibility that location-based attention also exists; they merely show that there is a contribution of objects per se in the allocation of attention.

Although the data from normal subjects suggest that at least one form of visual attention is allocated to objects, and so a pathological limitation of visual attention might well be a limitation in the number of objects attended, or in the ability to switch attention from object to object, regardless of the object's size or location, these data alone do not tell us anything about the neural basis of this visual attention process. In particular, they do not tell us whether the visual attention process that Posner has studied in parietal-damaged patients is object-based. The hypothesis that dorsal simultanagnosia consists of a bilateral "disengage" deficit would be strengthened if it turned out to be the case that parietal damage results in an inability to disengage attention from one *object* to a *different object* in the contralesional hemifield, as opposed to (or in addition to) from location to location. The critical experiments for answering this question have not been carried out. However, there are data available in answer to a highly similar question concerning neglect rather than the "disengage" deficit per se. Although Posner and colleagues have been careful not to equate neglect with a "disengage" deficit, the clinical manifestations of neglect certainly seem consistent with the inability of patients to disengage their attention for the perception of stimuli contralateral to their lesions, and many current discussions of these two conditions refer to them interchangeably. In fact, Morrow and Ratcliff (1988) have shown that there is a high correlation between neglect, as operationalized in terms of standard clinical tests such as line bisection and visual search, and the "disengage" deficit, as operationalized in Posner's lateralized cued simple reaction time task.

My colleagues and I have found that the structure of objects in central vision affects the distribution of attention in patients with neglect (Farah, Wallace, and Madigan, 1989), consistent with the hypothesis that the impaired visual attention system is object-based as well as location-based. We presented patients with a visual search task in which letters of the alphabet were scattered randomly over a page, and subjects were instructed to read all of the letters they could see. In addition to the letters on each page, there were two bloblike shapes, each about three times longer than wide, arranged in one of two ways: Either oriented horizonally and placed one above the other, straddling midline, or oriented vertically and placed one on each side of the page. Our subjects, who had right hemisphere damage and therefore left neglect, often started reading on the right side of the page (in contrast to most normal subjects, who search left to right) and omitted letters on the left. However, they started on the left more often, and read more letters on the left, when the two shapes straddled midline than when each was contained within a hemifield. This implies that the attentional process impaired in neglect is allocated not solely to locations, which were constant in the two conditions of this experiment, but also to objects, such that an object that is perceived in the hemifield ipsilateral to the lesion will have attention allocated to its entirety, even if it extends into the contralateral visual field. Brunn and Farah (in press) demonstrated that objects defined by more abstract properties can also affect the distribution of attention in neglect. We presented left neglect patients with word and nonword letter strings in central vision and assessed the distribution of attention in two ways: By having patients bisect lines drawn directly underneath the letter strings, and by having patients name the colors of the individual letters in the letter strings (which were printed in different colored inks). Patients bisected the lines more symmetrically, and named the colors on the left more accurately, when the letter strings were words than when they were nonwords. Thus, in neglect attention is allocated to objects defined by familiarity or recognizability, as well as low-level physical features. This is a further parallel between neglect (assumed here to reflect a unilateral disengage deficit) and the attentional limitation in dorsal simultanagnosia, in which whole meaningful objects such as words are perceived, regardless of size or complexity.

The finding that the "fracture lines" of attentional impairment following either unilateral or bilateral dorsal visual system damage are influenced by the boundaries of objects might seem puzzling, given what we know about the division of labor between the dorsal and ventral visual systems. It is supposed to be the ventral visual system that represents objects, and the dorsal system that is concerned solely with spatial location. Do the object-based attention effects observed in dorsal simultanagnosia, as well as in hemispatial neglect, imply that the parietal lobe represents objects, including objects defined by such abstract knowledge-dependent properties as lexicality? No, it simply implies that parietal-based attentional processes are part of an interactive system including other parts of the brain that do recognize objects and words. A possible account of how these different parts of the system might interact is sketched out in chapter 6.

3.2.3 Attention, visual disorientation, and the coding of spatial relations within and between objects

Although it is possible that visual disorientation is a separate disorder from the attentional limitation just discussed, the apparently perfect correlation that exists between these two disorders raises the possibility that they are different manifestations of the same underlying impairment. One plausible view of the relation between the two disorders is that visual disorientation is secondary to, and an inevitable consequence of, the attentional disorder in dorsal simultanagnosia. This is because the location of an object can only be specified relative to another location, be it the subject's finger (in a pointing task), another object (when describing the location), or the origin of some abstract coordinate system. The inability of dorsal simultanagnosics to attend to two separate loci would therefore be expected to impair localization. The introspection of one of Holmes's (1918) patients is consistent with this hypothesis. When asked to describe the relative positions of two objects placed side by side, one above the other, or one nearer to him, the patient made many errors and spontaneously explained his performance by saying that "I can only look at one at a time" (p. 453). An objection to this hypothesis comes from a thought experiment in which one imagines only being able to see one object at a time, for example, sitting in a dark room seeing one stimulus after another flashed on a blank screen. It doesn't seem as if this would induce visual disorientation, because one could simply keep track of the locations of the previous stimuli while perceiving the current stimulus. However, this "keeping track of" previous locations presumably involves allocating attention to them, something that dorsal simultanagnosics cannot do.

The issue of whether the ability to represent visual location and the ability to attend to visual stimuli are in principle separable has been more fully explored in discussions of neglect. One research tradition explains neglect in terms of an impairment of attentional processing affecting the contralesional side of space (e.g., Posner et al., 1984), whereas another postulates an impaired internal representation of the contralesional side of space (e.g., Bisiach, Luzzatti, and Perani, 1979). However, it has been argued that these explanations are perfectly compatible, differing only in emphasis (Farah, Wong, Monheit, and Morrow, 1989; Shallice, 1988, chapter 13). Attention is not allocated to objects at locations in space, but rather to internal representations of objects at locations in space. Therefore, even according to an attentional account, neglect involves internal representations of the contralesional hemispace that cannot be used normally. Likewise, because attention operates on representations, a representational account of neglect implies that attention cannot be deployed in the contralesional hemispace. The same arguments apply to the bilateral impairment of location representation and attention in dorsal simultanagnosia.

The impairment of spatial representation in dorsal simultanagnosia, whatever its relation to attentional impairments, poses an interesting paradox when contrasted with the preservation of shape perception in this syndrome. After all, shape is nothing but the spatial relations among the parts of an object, or at the finest level of resolution, among the points in space occupied by the object. Yet as impaired as dorsal simultanagnosics are in their ability to perceive the spatial relations among objects, they are almost invariably normal in their ability to recognize objects on the basis of shape. Their very occasional difficulties in object recognition occur because they have not *seen* the entirety of the object, in the sense of simply detecting that other parts of the object are present. It is worth noting that their ability to copy shapes is a misleading measure of their ability to perceive them. These patients are generally unable to copy drawings that they have recognized easily, and their attempts at copying have a characteristic "exploded" look, like the drawing of a bicycle shown in figure 13. This can be understood in terms of the necessity, in copying a picture, for drawing a part at a time, which requires patients to shift their attention to the individual parts of the shape and to position the parts with respect to one another. Of course, seeing multiple items and locating them with respect to one another is precisely what dorsal simultanagnosics cannot do. The patient whose copy is shown in figure 13 put it thus: "As soon as I lift my pencil from the paper I can't see what I have drawn and have to guess where to put the next detail" (Godwin-Austen, 1965, p. 455). Copying is not the straightforward test of shape perception that it might, at first glance, seem to be. This point will arise again in the next chapter, in the form of the opposite dissociation: good copies and impaired perception.

The discrepancy between normal perception of shape and impaired perception of spatial relations among objects is only paradoxical if one assumes that spatial relations within an object are coded by the visual system in the same way as spatial relations between objects. A priori this would seem to be a very reasonable assumption. Indeed Kosslyn (1987) has proposed that the dorsal system's location representations are used to represent the spatial relations among the parts of objects during object recognition. However, the dissociation between these abililites in dorsal simultanagnosia implies that these two kinds of spatial information are

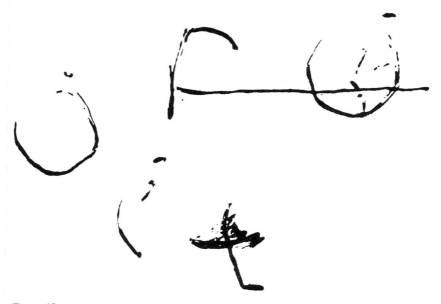

Figure 13
A copy of a bicycle made by a dorsal simultanagnosic patient who was able to recognize objects and drawings.

coded differently. The spatial relations among objects and the spatial relations among the parts of a single object seem to be represented by the visual system using different underlying mechanisms.

3.3 Ventral Simultanagnosia

Several rather explicit accounts have been offered of the underlying deficit in ventral simultanagnosia. Kinsbourne and Warrington (1962) took their data to imply that visual stimuli are recognized serially, and that in ventral simultanagnosics there is an abnormally long "refractory period" between acts of recognition. This conclusion was based on their findings of approximately normal tachistoscopic recognition thresholds for single items, and greatly elevated recognition thresholds for two or more items, even when presented sequentially. Warrington and Rabin (1971) later suggested that the impairment lies in visual short-term memory, because of the effect of familiarity of letter sequence (not a perceptual property) on the number of letters reported by these patients. Levine and Calvanio (1978) argue that the locus of impairment must be in the visual recognition per se of the stimuli, given their patients' poor performance on tasks with virtually no memory load. They also suggest that the impaired recognition process could not be occurring serially, as Kinsbourne and Warrington claimed, because this would imply that the similarity of flanking letters would have no effect on patients' ability to report a given letter, contrary to what they found. The interpretations offered above differ along two main dimensions: whether the locus of the deficit in ventral simultanagnosia is perceptual or postperceptual, and whether stimuli are (normally, and in ventral simultanagnosia) recognized serially or in parallel. Let us start with the first of these issues.

3.3.1 Perceptual or postperceptual bottleneck?
Warrington and Rabin (1971) were the first to point out that the processing limitation in ventral simultanagnosia is determined not only by the physical characteristics of the visual stimuli, but also by their familiarity: The more closely a sequence of letters approximates English, the more of the letters left-posterior-damaged patients can recognize in a given amount of time. Levine and Calvanio (1978) made similar observations, noting that more letters could be named by ventral simultanagnosics in words than in nonword letter strings. Because performance was being affected by properties of the stimuli that could not be called "perceptual" (such as brightness or complexity), but which have been related to stimulus memorability in many memory studies (e.g., Baddeley, 1964), Warrington and Rabin concluded that the locus of the effect must be postperceptual, and they identified visual short-term memory as a likely candidate. In the years since Warrington and Rabin made this argument, cognitive psychologists have found many examples of stimulus perception being facilitated by the familiarity or meaningfulness of the stimulus context (e.g., Biederman, 1972; Palmer, 1975; Reicher, 1969; Wheeler, 1970; Weisstein and Harris, 1974). The most thoroughly studied of these phenomena is the "word superiority effect," which refers to the fact that letters are perceived more quickly and accurately when embedded in a word than when presented alone or in a nonword. This facilitation from word context is not a result of postperceptual guessing, based on the assumption that the letter in question must make a word with the other letters, because it is observed in forced choice tasks when both choices would make a word (e.g., the second letter in the word "read" followed by the choices "e" and "o"). The effect is also found for pseudowords, which conform to the orthographic rules of the language, a condition similar to Warrington and Rabin's statistical approximations to English. Furthermore, progress has been made in understanding, mechanistically, how contextual familiarity could affect perceptual processing. McClelland and Rumelhart (1981) present a computational model that accounts in a simple and parsimonious way for most of the findings

concerning word superiority in letter perception. Figure 14 shows a schematic depiction of part of their model. Because of the importance of this issue to the interpretation of ventral simultanagnosia, a brief overview of the model will be offered here.

Letter units are initially activated by an amount proportional to the input they receive from the units representing their constituent features. The letter units then pass activation on to the words with which they are consistent. For example, if there appears to be a "t" in the first position, that will cause the words "trap," "trip," "take," and "time" to gain activation. In addition, word units are inhibited by the activation of units that are inconsistent with the word. For example, "able" will be inhibited by the unit representing an initial "t," as activation in these units represents incompatible hypotheses, and "able" will also be inhibited by activation in other word units for the same reason. So far, this model would seem to account for word recognition, but it is not yet clear how it accounts for the word superiority effect, nor is it clear how it accounts for phenomena involving pseudowords, that is, statistical approximations to real words. The word superiority effect is explained by postulating feedback from the word level to the letter level. Switching to a different set of examples from those shown in figure 14, if the word shown is "read," and perception of the letter in the second position is just barely adequate, so that the "e" unit is ever so slightly more activated than the "o" unit, then this will give the edge to the word "read" over the word "road." Inter-word inhibition will then drive the activation of the "road" unit down, and feedback from the word level to the letter level

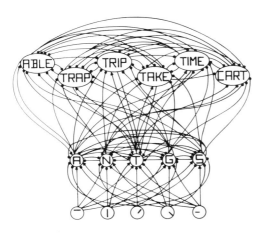

Figure 14
Part of the McClelland and Rumelhart interactive activation model of letter and word perception. See text for an explanation.

will therefore consist of greater "top-down" support for "e" than for "o." Thus, people will be more accurate at discriminating "e" from "o" in the context of "read" than in a nonword context or alone. Why should pseudowords also give rise to superior letter perception, given that there are no units corresponding to them at the word level? Because pseudowords are sufficiently similar to real words that their constituent letters will at least partially activate some real word units. "yead," for example, will activate "year," "bead," "read," and so on. Once these word units have become activated, they will inhibit other word units that are less consistent with the activated letter level units, and will provide top-down support for the letters that do occur in the words similar to "yead," including, for example, the "e" in the second position.

The implication of this work on the word superiority effect is that the familiarity effects observed by Warrington and Rabin and Levine and Calvanio are perfectly consistent with a perceptual locus for the underlying deficit in ventral simultanagnosia. In addition, there are data which suggest that the deficit is perceptual and not postperceptual: For example, the finding of Levine and Calvanio that location precues facilitate performance but postcues do not. Therefore, it seems correct to conclude that the ventral simultanagnosics have difficulty in the perceptual recognition of multiple stimuli.

3.3.2 Parallel or serial recognition of multiple stimuli?

The second issue on which accounts of ventral simultanagnosia differ is whether or not multiple stimuli are normally recognized serially or in parallel. Kinsbourne and Warrington (1962) suggest that in normal subjects and in their brain-damaged subjects, recognition proceeds serially, based on the equivalence of simultaneous and sequential stimulus presentation. Levine and Calvanio (1978) argue that certain aspects of their data (e.g., effects of similarity of flanking letters) imply parallel processing. In fact, research in cognitive psychology, reported after Kinsbourne and Warrington's (1962) paper, has suggested that small numbers of familiar forms are normally recognized in parallel. Most of this research is designed to contrast visual search performance for a particular "target" letter or digit under conditions in which all stimuli are visible at once, and when the stimulus set is presented in two separate, sequential observation intervals, each one as long as the interval in the single presentation condition (e.g., Eriksen and Spencer, 1969; Shiffrin and Gardner, 1972; Pashler and Badgio, 1987). If subjects recognize the characters serially, then they should benefit from the additional time *per character* available in the sequential presentation condition. In contrast, if subjects recognize the characters in parallel, independent channels, then performance in the two conditions should be equivalent. The findings imply parallel processing.[1] Converging evidence for parallel processing comes from the work of Pashler and Badgio (1985), showing that the effect of stimulus degradation (which presumably affects the visual recognition process) is additive, rather than interactive, with the effect of the number of items to be recognized.

According to the parallel recognition hypothesis, what is the nature of the processing deficit in ventral simultanagnosia? One possibility that accounts for the data currently at hand is that there has been a reduction of the normal amount of processing capacity, such that enough capacity remains for the normal recognition of a single stimulus, but there is insufficient capacity left for recognizing two or more stimuli. This account would explain Levine and Calvanio's results in the following way: When patients are precued with the location of the stimulus to be recognized, they can devote their entire processing capacity to that stimulus. When recognizing or performing "same/different" matching on multiple stimuli, the shortage of processing capacity may result in morphological errors due to incomplete analysis of the stimulus: calling an "N" a "W," or saying that the string "OCO" is made up of identical letters. Similarly, the poorer performance at recognizing complex rather than simple letters is consistent with capacity limitations.

Levine and Calvanio (1978) argue against a capacity limitation based on the preserved ability of ventral simultanagnosics to recognize faces. They point out that a single face is far more complex, and more similar to other stimuli of its kind, than a single letter, and yet a single face does not overly tax these patients' processing capacity. However, the intuitive metrics of complexity and similarity being used in this argument may not be the relevant ones for understanding the information-processing limitations of object recognition. The speed and accuracy with which normal subjects encode, retain over long periods, and later recognize faces, compared to other stimuli, does nothing to support the view that faces are especially taxing stimuli for our object recognition systems. The extent to which a stimulus will tax object recognition capacity will surely depend on the accessibility of the stored representations of the object and on the distinctiveness of those representations with respect to other similar representations. Evidence from single unit recording in monkeys, to be described in section 5.2.2, suggests that the primate brain has devoted a great deal of representational machinery to the representation of faces. Therefore, faces may be no more taxing of object recognition capacity than other apparently simpler stimuli, such as letters.[2] A more appropriate comparison for assessing the effects of complexity on the ability of ventral simultanagnosics to recognize stimuli would be between more and less complex stimuli of a single kind, such as letters. Consistent with a capacity limitation, Levine and Calvanio (1982) note that *groups* of simple letters (i.e., few line segments) are better perceived by ventral simultanagnosics than groups of complex letters.

Another apparent problem with the parallel limited capacity view is that it seems rather coincidental that recognition capacity would be reduced to just the level needed to recognize a single item more or less normally, but not multiple items. Why wouldn't capacity sometimes be reduced to a level above or below that needed for one item? In fact, there is evidence that it often is. Patients who have difficulty recognizing single items must technically be excluded by definition from the category "simultanagnosia," but in fact some ventral simultanagnosics make occasional errors in recognizing even single stimuli, and there is often an evolution in the course of recovery in left posterior-damaged patients from a state in which single items are frequently misidentified to a state in which they meet the exclusionary defining criteria of ventral simultanagnosia (Levine and Calvanio, 1982). Indeed, Kinsbourne and Warrington say that they view simultanagnosia as part of a continuum of disorders, bordered on the more impaired side by "those severe cases of disorder known as visual object agnosia [i.e. single objects cannot be recognized]" and on the normal side by "patients with minor or residual damage to the dominant occipital lobe who have escaped clinical detection altogether; perhaps their speed of reading is slowed up, but no more" (p. 483). Consistent with this idea of a continuum, the four patients in Kinsbourne and Warrington's (1962) study differed in the severity of their disorder, requiring different exposure durations to obtain comparable levels of performance. In chapters 4 and 5 we will discuss patients who, it will be argued, have the same underlying problem as those labelled "simultanagnosics" by Kinsbourne, Warrington, Levine, and Calvanio, and whose degrees of impairment span a wide range.

A final remark on the relation between ventral simultanagnosia and object recognition is that "capacity" is one of the less satisfying explanatory terms in psychology. Therefore, the hypothesis that ventral simultanagnosia consists of a reduction in the processing capacity of a parallel recognition system is probably better viewed as a general class of hypotheses, which await more mechanistic formulations and empirical tests.

3.4 Perceptual Categorization Deficit

An influential framework for interpreting impairments in object recognition has been put forth by Warrington (e.g., Warrington and Taylor, 1978; Warrington, 1982, 1985). In this framework, diagrammed in figure 15, there are two major stages in object recognition, one carried out by each hemisphere. The existence and nature of the first stage, "perceptual

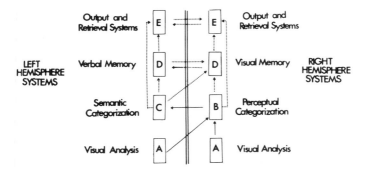

Figure 15
Warrington and Taylor's model of visual object recognition.

categorization," was based on Warrington's observations of right-parietal-damaged patients, who are impaired at recognizing and matching objects photographed at unconventional perspectives or under uneven lighting and are, in Warrington's terms, apperceptive agnosics. This stage is hypothesized to involve the extraction of a viewpoint-invariant shape representation from the two-dimensional representation of an object yielded by early visual processing in the occipital lobes. A second stage, localized in the posterior left hemisphere, was postulated on the basis of Warrington's observations of patients with "semantic categorization deficits," whom she refers to as "associative agnosics." This syndrome will be discussed in chapters 4 and 5. According to Warrington, in the "semantic categorization" stage, the representation constructed by the right parietal lobe in the course of "perceptual categorization" is associated with semantic knowledge about the object.

3.4.1 Mechanisms of perceptual categorization
Several specific hypotheses have been put forth concerning the nature of the visual processes that have been impaired in patients with perceptual categorization deficit. These hypotheses are of interest not only for what they tell us about the state of these patients' perceptual abilities. If a process can be selectively impaired, this argues for the existence of that process in the first place, and hence evidence concerning the specific processes that have been disrupted in patients with perceptual categorization deficit stands to tell us about the processes underlying normal perceptual categorization.

Marr (1982) theorized that object recognition depends upon the construction of an object-centered representation of shape, that is, a description of the object's shape with respect to a coordinate system centered on the object. The computational advantage of such representations is that they automatically yield the various shape constancies. This is because as the object changes its position, size, or orientation, so does the object-centered coordinate system, and descriptions of the object's shape with respect to that coordinate system are therefore constant over these changes. The computational disadvantage of object-centered representations is that they are difficult to derive from the stimulus image because one must assign the object-centered coordinate system before knowing what the object is. Marr suggested that certain low-level physical cues in the image, such as axes of elongation or symmetry, could guide the assignment of the appropriate coordinate system. He therefore interpreted the difficulty of right-posteriorly-damaged patients as an impairment in the ability to assign an object-centered frame of reference to a stimulus when the most salient cues to the proper orientation of the object-centered coordinate system, namely axes of elongation, were distorted by the foreshortening that generally results from unconventional perspectives.

Humphreys and Riddoch (1984, 1985) argued that there are two routes to perceptual categorization: one involves assigning an object-centered coordinate system, as Marr (1982) suggested, and the other involves noticing the characteristic and relatively viewpoint-invariant features of the object. They supported this claim with the case studies reviewed in the last chapter, in which a small group of right-hemisphere-damaged patients were found to be more impaired at recognizing foreshortened views than views showing minimal features, whereas a bilateral associative agnosic patient showed the opposite trend. These findings certainly indicate that foreshortening is more detrimental to the right hemisphere patients than minimizing the characteristic features, at least in the stimulus set used by Humphreys and Riddoch. The issue of whether there is a double dissociation between the performance of the two types of patient on the two types of stimulus is beset by statistical problems related to the small stimulus set (see Humphreys and Riddoch, 1985), and for reasons discussed by Shallice (1988) it is probably premature to conclude that the performance of H.J.A. represents a selective impairment of feature-based perceptual categorization.

The hypothesis that the right posterior perceptual categorization deficit is caused by an impairment in deriving an object-centered coordinate system from the retinotopic image was endorsed by Marr on computational grounds, and is consistent with the data of Humphreys and Riddoch (1984). However, the recent findings of Warrington and James (1986) call this hypothesis into question. Recall that these researchers created silhouettes of objects by back-illuminating them, rotating them from an initially unconventional perspective into a conventional perspective. Although they found that the right-hemisphere-damaged patients required more rotation towards the conventional perspective before recognizing the objects than the normal control subjects, consistent with a perceptual categorization deficit, they did no worse when the objects were initially foreshortened than when the axis of elongation was preserved. Reasoning by elimination, Warrington and James suggested that because the perceptual categorization deficit seems insensitive to manipulations designed to affect the assignment of object-centered coordinate systems, it might be better conceptualized in terms of impaired feature extraction. This conclusion seems to conflict with the findings of Humphreys and Riddoch (1984), who found that minimizing the visible features of objects did not impair the performance of their right-hemisphere-damaged patients, but that foreshortening did. Warrington and James (1986, p. 365) suggest a possible reinterpretation of Humphreys and Riddoch's data, according to which both kinds of unconventional views used by Humphreys and Riddoch involved the "radical" alteration of a major axis, and the good performance of Humphreys and Riddoch's right-hemisphere-damaged patients on one of the two types of unconventional views therefore shows that, in fact, these patients too were "not impaired." Unless it is being claimed that, in fact, the minimal feature views of Humphreys and Riddoch involved relatively *more* distortion of major axes than the foreshortened views, and/or their foreshortened views involved more minimization of featural information than the minimal feature views, it is not clear how the findings of Humphreys and Riddoch can be accommodated within Warrington and James's (1986) hypothesis. One possibility is that the two research groups were studying different kinds of impairment. This is plausible given that Warrington and James's subjects were an unselected group of consecutively admitted right-hemisphere-damaged patients, whereas Humphreys and Riddoch's subjects were selected for their poor performance on tests of unconventional views.

At present, the ratio of critical data to hypotheses is probably too low to expect any immediate resolution of these issues. Only recently have researchers attempted to discriminate empirically between different processes underlying the recognition of unconventional views (i.e., Humphreys and Riddoch, 1984; Warrington and James, 1986), and they have used different patient populations and different ways of operationalizing axis-based and feature-based processing. In addition, the set of hypotheses under consideration has so far been limited to those involving unconventional perspectives, even though earlier findings (Warrington and Ackroyd unpublished data, cited by Warrington 1982, 1985) suggest that the underlying impairment extends to recognition of objects viewed under uneven illumination, and perhaps even to pictures and symbols that are fragmented or incomplete (Warrington, 1982, 1985).

3.4.2 Role of "perceptual categorization" in normal object recognition

In addition to considering different hypotheses about the processes underlying performance in perceptual categorization tasks, and devising empirical tests capable of distinguishing among them, we should also ask a more fundamental question: Do these tasks have anything to do with normal object recognition? A salient feature of patients with so-called perceptual categorization deficit is that they show no impairment in recognizing objects in normal life. Furthermore, normal subjects often require a few seconds to view the "unconventional views" photographs before they hazard a recognition response (personal observation), and their performance is not error-free (e.g, Humphreys and Riddoch, 1984; Warrington and Taylor, 1973). It may therefore be more reasonable to view the perceptual categorization tasks as a kind of visual problem-solving rather than as an instance of visual object recognition proper. Indeed, in a recent paper Warrington and James (1988) state that "we would now wish to argue that perceptual categorization systems may be an optional resource rather than an obligatory stage of visual analysis," contrasting with earlier suggestions that the ability tapped by their perceptual categorization tasks represents one of two major stages in normal visual object recognition (see figure 15).

The view that the right hemisphere patients' deficit in perceptual categorization tasks should not be considered an impairment in object recognition ability per se, but an impairment only for the perception of stimuli made artificially difficult to see, is consistent with results from lateral tachistoscopic studies of normal subjects. These studies have suggested a special role for the right hemisphere in the perception of visual stimuli that have been degraded in any number of ways, including brightness reduction, contrast reduction, size reduction, reduction of exposure duration, and blurring (Michimata and Hellige, 1987; Sergent and Hellige, 1986). Although this interpretation leaves unanswered the question of what process or processes allow the right hemisphere to cope with this variety of types of visual degradation, it does suggest that the right hemisphere's contribution to object recognition, observed in tasks such as recognizing unconventional views, may come into play *only* in such tasks.

Chapter 4
The Associative Agnosias

Like the term "apperceptive agnosia," "associative agnosia" has been used quite broadly to cover a heterogeneous set of conditions. These include impairments in general semantic knowledge not confined to the visual modality and impairments confined to the naming (as opposed to the recognition) of visually presented objects. Associative agnosia is also often taken to be a more specific syndrome, in which patients have a selective impairment in the recognition of visually presented objects, despite apparently adequate visual perception of them. It is with this narrower sense of associative agnosia that we will begin.

4.1 Associative Visual Object Agnosia (Narrow Sense)

There are three criteria for membership in this category. The first is difficulty recognizing a variety of visually presented objects, as demonstrated by naming as well as such nonverbal tests of recognition as grouping objects together according to their semantic category or gesturing to indicate their normal functions. The second criterion is normal recognition of objects through modalities other than vision, for example by touching the object, hearing its characteristic sound, or being given a verbal definition of it.[1] The third criterion is intact visual perception, or at least visual perception that seems adequate to the task of recognizing the object. This last criterion is usually tested by having patients copy objects or drawings that they cannot recognize, or match pairs of such stimuli as being the same or different.

A well-documented case of associative object agnosia was reported by Rubens and Benson in 1971. Their subject was a middle-aged man who had suffered an acute loss of blood pressure with resulting brain damage. His mental status and language abilities were normal, and his visual acuity was 20/30, with a right homonymous hemianopia (blindness in the right visual hemifield). His one severe impairment was an inability to recognize most visual stimuli.

For the first three weeks in the hospital the patient could not identify common objects presented visually and did not know what was on his plate until he tasted it. He identified objects immediately on touching them. When shown a stethoscope, he described it as "a long cord with a round thing at the end," and asked if it could be a watch. He identified a can opener as "could be a key." Asked to name a cigarette lighter, he said, "I don't know" but named it after the examiner lit it. He said he was "not sure" when shown a toothbrush. Asked to identify a comb, he said, "I don't know." When shown a large matchbook, he said, "It could be a container for keys." He correctly identifed glasses. For a pipe, he said, "Some type of utensil, I'm not sure." Shown a key, he said, "I don't know what that is; perhaps a file or a tool of some sort."

He was never able to describe or demonstrate the use of an object if he could not name it. If he misnamed an object his demonstration of its use would correspond to the mistaken identification. Identification improved very slightly when given the category of the object (e.g., "something to eat") or when asked to point to a named object instead of being required to give the name. When told the correct name of an object, he usually responded with a quick nod and said, "Yes, I see it now." Then, often he could point out various parts of the previously unrecognized item as readily as a normal subject (e.g., the stem and bowl of a pipe, and the laces, sole, and heel of a shoe). However, if asked by the examiner "Suppose I told you that the last object was not really a pipe, what would you say?" He would reply, "I would take your word for it. Perhaps it's not really a pipe." Similar vacillation never occurred with tactilely or aurally identified objects.

After three weeks on the ward, object naming ability had improved so that he could name many common objects, but this was variable; he might correctly name an object one time and misname it later. Performance deteriorated severely if any part of the object was covered by the examiner. He could match identical objects but not group objects by categories (clothing, food). He could draw the outlines of objects (key, spoon, etc.) which he could not identify.

He was unable to recognize members of his family, the hospital staff, or even his own face in the mirror . . . Sometimes he had difficulty distinguishing a line drawing of an animal's face from a man's face, but he always recognized it as a face.

Ability to recognize pictures of objects was greatly impaired, and after repeated testing he could name only one or two out of ten line drawings. He was always able to name geometrical forms (circle, square, triangle, cube). Remarkably, he could make excellent copies of line drawings and still fail to name the subject . . . He easily matched drawings of objects that he could not identify, and had no difficulty discriminating between complex nonrepresentational patterns differing from each other only subtly. He occasionally failed in discriminating because he included imperfections in the paper or in the printer's ink. He could never group drawings by class unless he could first name the subject.

Reading, both aloud and for comprehension, was greatly limited. He could read, hesitantly, most printed letters, but often misread "K" as "R" and "L" as "T" and vice versa . . . He was able to read words slowly by spelling them aloud. (pp. 308–309)

In Rubens and Benson's case, we see all of the elements of associative object agnosia: Impaired visual object recognition demonstrated verbally and nonverbally, intact recognition of objects through other modalities, and evidence from drawing tasks and matching tasks suggesting that perception was sufficient to allow recognition. Other well-known cases that meet these criteria of associative visual object agnosia include Albert, Reches, and Silverberg (1975); Bauer (1982); Davidoff and Wilson (1985); Hecaen and Ajuriaguerra (1956); Levine (1978); Levine and Calvanio (1989); Mack and Boller (1977); Macrae and Trolle (1956); McCarthy and Warrington (1986), Pillon, Signoret, and Lhermitte (1981); Ratcliff and Newcombe (1982); Riddoch and Humphreys (1987); and Wapner, Judd, and Gardner (1978). Many other cases are listed in table 1 of chapter 5. Figures 1, 16, and 17 show examples of the impressive ability possessed by some of these patients to copy drawings, even when they could not recognize what it was that they were copying.

Although the perceptual abilities of these patients with associative agnosia are quite good compared to the apperceptive agnosics described earlier, there are some indications that their perception is not normal. Furthermore, there are even some indications that these perceptual impairments play a causal role in the difficulties that associative agnosic patients have with visual object recognition. Let us examine the different kinds of evidence that have been taken to be relevant to the status of perception in associative agnosia.

Traditionally, the ability to render a recognizable copy of a stimulus was considered an appropriate test of patients' ability to *see* a recognizable percept of the stimulus. Thus, these patients were described as seeing "a normal percept, stripped of its meaning" (Teuber, 1968). At first glance, this seems a reasonable inference to make. However, Levine (1978) points out that "accurate drawings can be produced despite impaired visual perception. A patient who can see in any single visual fixation only one or two features of a complex visual pattern may nevertheless . . . produce sequentially what he cannot perceive simultaneously" (p. 363). The other primary source of evidence for intact perception in associative agnosia is the ability to match a stimulus with the identical stimulus in a set of similar-looking stimuli. As with copying, accurate matching can be accomplished when perception is abnormal, using feature-by-feature matching, verbal mediation, or any number of other special strategies.

In general, the more carefully investigators have examined visual perception in these cases, the more abnormal it has been revealed to be. These abnormalities have shown up in a wide range of different kinds of tests, and it is not yet clear whether they all represent the impairment of a single kind of underlying visual process or whether qualitatively different perceptual impairments are implicated in different cases of associative agnosia. Nevertheless, the simple generalization that associative agnosics have intact perception is called into question by a variety of findings, which will be summarized here.

The possibility raised by Levine (1978) that normal-looking drawings might be the product of abnormal perception with compensatory copying strategies seems to be confirmed by the available data. In the cases in which the patient's manner of copying has been described, it has been reported to be abnormal. For example, although Rubens and Benson did not themselves describe their patient's manner of copying the drawings shown in figure 1, Brown (1972, p. 216), who observed the patient during the same time as Rubens and Benson, describes the patient's copying ability as "fairly accurate but slavish." Ratcliff and Newcombe (1982) describe patient M.S.'s copies (see figure 16) as "remarkably accurate, although they appear to be achieved through a line by line copying strategy" (p. 161). The copies made by patient L.H. (described by Levine and Calvanio, 1989), shown in figure 17, were executed exceedingly slowly, with one or two lines drawn at a time, and with many long pauses to inspect the original drawings and to compare them with the copy being made. Humphreys and Riddoch (1987a) show an impressive copy made by patient H.J.A. of an etching of St. Paul's Cathedral and note that it took him six hours to complete! Levine (1978) reports that patient F.Z. proceeded slowly when copying, and often lost her place if she took her pen off the paper. Wapner, Judd, and Gardner (1978) describe their patient's manner of copying as "slavish," and note that this patient, too, would often lose his place in the middle of a drawing, resulting in carefully rendered pictures of such anomalies as a five-legged rhinoceros or an accordion with three keyboards.

As with drawing tasks, the manner in which associative agnosics perform matching tasks appears to be abnormal, even when the end

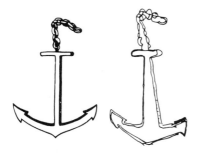

Figure 16
Copy of an anchor made by patient M.S., who was unable to recognize the anchor.

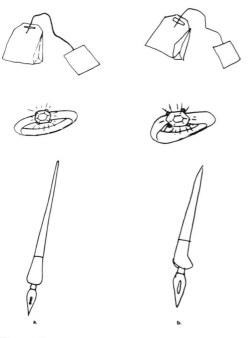

a.   b.

Figure 17
Copies of a teabag, ring, and pen made by patient L.H., who was unable to recognize the drawings he had copied.

result is good. The observation of Rubens and Benson that their patient tended to mistake imperfections in the paper or printer's ink for differences in the pattern suggests that he was not performing the task as normal subjects would. In addition, we do not know how complex or similar to one another these patterns were. Performance on matching tasks is not informative unless we know how different the patterns being compared are. Although Levine's patient F.Z. performed well on simple matching tasks, she did poorly when the patterns were complex and differed only subtly from each other.

Many authors have noted that associative agnosics are highly sensitive to the perceptual quality of the stimulus, an observation which is at least consistent with impaired visual perception in these patients. In general, objects are easiest for these patients to identify, followed by photographs and then line drawings (e.g., Boudouresques, Poncet, Sebahoun, and Alicherif, 1972, case 1; Cambier, Masson, Elghozi, Henin, and Viader, 1980; Levine and Calvanio, 1989; Mack and Boller, 1977; Ratcliff and Newcombe, 1982; Riddoch and Humphreys, 1987a; Rubens and Benson, 1971), an ordering that reflects increasing impoverishment of the stimulus. Rubens and Benson noted that occlusion of part of an object caused great difficulty for their patient, and some authors have found that the performance of associative agnosics drops sharply with tachistoscopic presentation of stimuli (e.g., Levine, 1978; Macrae and Trolle, 1956; Cole and Perez-Cruet, 1964).

Similarly, when the errors made by associative agnosic patients have been analyzed, "visual errors," that is, misidentifying an object as a similar looking object, are reported to be common (e.g., Boudouresques, et al., 1972, case 1; Cambier et al., 1980; Davidoff and Wilson, 1985; Levine, 1978; Mack and Boller, 1977; Newcombe and Ratcliff, 1974; Ratcliff and Necombe, 1982; Rubens and Benson's, 1971, case as described by Brown, 1972). Levine (1978) recorded the responses of patient F.Z. to 300 consecutive objects and pictures of objects and classified them as either correct, visually similar in overall form, visually similar by virtue of a shared feature, perseveration, no response, and "other." The patient was correct on 80 of the trials, made no response on 39, named an object that was visually similar in overall form on 51 trials, and named an object that was visually similar by virtue of a common feature on 33 trials. The remainder of the responses were either perseverative or bore no relation to the stimulus. Thus, the majority of errors were visual in nature. This tally agrees well with my observations of the associative agnosic L.H. For example, he misidentified a drawing of a baseball bat on four different occasions, and each time his answer was a different object of similar shape: a paddle, a knife, a baster, and a thermometer. Davidoff and Wilson (1985) describe an associative agnosic patient, J.R., who makes both visual and semantic errors in object recognition, but report that the semantic errors can be eliminated by narrowing the choice of alternative responses, whereas the visual errors cannot. When asked to point to a named object from a set of drawn objects, she sometimes chose a visually dissimilar but semantically related item (e.g., trumpet for violin, a semantic error), or a semantically unrelated but visually similar item (e.g., hose for measuring tape, a visual error). When the authors then offered the patient a forced choice between her error and the correct choice, the semantic errors were reduced but the visual errors were intractable.

Some very recent studies of associative agnosia have included special tasks designed to assess visual perception with more sensitivity than the traditional drawing, matching, and tachistoscopic tasks described earlier. For example, Ratcliff and Newcombe (1982) presented patient M.S. with "possible" and "impossible" figures of the kind shown in figure 18. Although his perception seemed normal by the criterion of his finished copies of drawings (see figure 16), he was unable to distinguish possible from impossible figures. More recently, Ratcliff (unpublished work) has related this finding to M.S.'s laborious, line-by-line drawing strategy by comparing the amount of time taken to copy possible and impossible figures by normal subjects and by this patient. Whereas normal subjects are considerably faster in copying the "possible" figures, presumably because the overall structure of the figure can guide them, patient M.S. requires the same amount of time to copy both types of figure, as if he were not able to be guided by the structure of the "possible" figures.

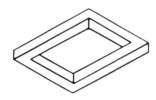

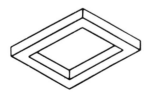

Figure 18
Example of an impossible figure (top) and a possible figure (bottom).

Riddoch and Humphreys (1987a) describe a patient, H.J.A., whose pattern of performance on classical tests for associative agnosia would place him squarely among the cases of "normal perception, stripped of its meaning," but who, on closer examination, shows impaired visual perception. H.J.A. was disproportionately impaired, relative to normal subjects, at recognizing overlapping drawings, a task which the authors argue particularly taxes visual segmentation processes. He was also paradoxically better at recognizing objects that were depicted in silhouette than as line drawings, suggesting to the authors that something was amiss with his ability to perceive or integrate the details of a visual stimulus. Humphreys and Riddoch (1987a) briefly describe the results of feature integration experiments with H.J.A. Their basic task consists of deciding whether or not an upside-down "T" is present among a set of upright "T"s. This task is classified as a feature integration task by Humphreys and Riddoch because in order to discriminate an upright from an upside-down "T" one must correctly integrate the vertical and horizontal contour features of the letters. When these stimuli are arranged in a circle, normal subjects seem to be able to use the overall configuration of the stimulus display to facilitate their decision: In the "absent" condition, in which the display has a "good" configuration (in the gestalt psychology sense), normal subjects are extremely fast and their response times depend only very weakly on the number of stimulus letters in the display. In contrast, when the letters are arranged randomly, the "absent" responses of normal subjects are no faster than their "present" responses, and show the same degree of dependence on the number of letters in the display as the "present" responses. H.J.A.'s pattern of response times were the same whether the stimulus display is arranged in a circle or randomly: He never shows the fast "absent" response. Humphreys and Riddoch interpret this as a sign of difficulty with feature integration. It is also interesting from the point of view of configurational processing, as this is the distinguishing property of the condition in which H.J.A.'s feature integration performance differed qualitatively from that of normal subjects.

Mendez (1988) and Levine and Calvanio (1989) assessed the visual perception of associative agnosic patients using a variety of tasks tapping different aspects of visual and spatial ability. Mendez found that his two cases performed adequately on simple visual tests (e.g., Benton Line Orientation test, Benton Visual Form Discrimination test) and on a test of mental rotation ability, but were both impaired on tests that emphasized gestalt perception of stimuli presented in fragmented or masked form (Hooper Visual Organization test, Southern California Integration Test and the Gestalt Completion test; see Lezak, 1983, for descriptions of the aforementioned tests).

Levine and Calvanio (1989) arrived at similar conclusions in their testing of patient L.H. with the factor-analyzed test kit of Ekstrom, French and Harman (1976). They found that most of the perceptual factors measured in the test battery were reasonably preserved in L.H.: He fell somewhere between above average and mildly impaired on tests measuring the "visual-verbal closure" factor, the "flexibility of visual closure" factor, the "spatial orientation" factor, and the "spatial scanning" factor. Visual-verbal closure refers to the ability to identify a printed word when some of the letters are missing, scrambled, or embedded in other letters. Flexibility of closure refers to the ability to resist closure and is tapped by tasks that involve finding a previously given geometric shape when it is part of another well-defined shape. Spatial orientation ability is tapped by mental rotation tests, in which the subject must decide whether two objects or patterns are the same despite different orientations. Finally, spatial scanning is the ability to find paths through complex mazes. L.H.'s performance on tests of the "perceptual speed" factor, which require rapid comparisons between figures and rapid visual search for a prespecified target figure, was rated moderately to severely impaired. However, the authors note that he was highly accurate in these tasks, raising the possibility that he might have performed better if pushed to go faster. In contrast to these relatively preserved perceptual abilities, L.H. was severely impaired on the tests that tap "visual closure," the ability to perceive the shape and identity of an object that has been fragmented or degraded by visual noise. Note that the difference between the visual closure factor and the visual-verbal closure factor is not simply a difference between nonverbal and verbal visual stimuli: One of the tests that loads on the visual closure factor, and on which L.H. did very poorly, involves recognizing words that have been fragmented (the "concealed words" test). In this test the fragmentation of the words does not leave the component letters intact, but fragments the overall pattern of the word without regard to letter boundaries. Figure 19 shows examples of items that test visual closure.

The introspections of associative agnosics are also consistent with perceptual abnormalities. For example, Levine's (1978) patient admitted to "blurriness" in her vision (p. 353). Wapner et al's (1978) patient frequently complained that "everything seemed dim, as if it were twilight" and also remarked "I have to use my mind to interpret what I'm seeing. My eyes used to do that" (p. 347). Rubens and Benson's (1971) patient complained that faces seemed "out of focus, almost as though a haze were in front of them" (p. 308).

Given the evidence for impaired visual perception in associative agnosics, is there any reason to distinguish between apperceptive and

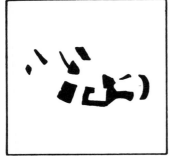

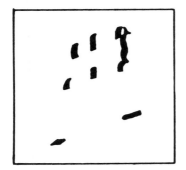

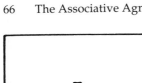

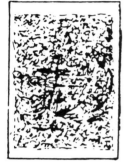

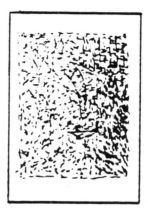

Figure 19
Examples of stimuli that test different forms of "closure" ability, in which patient L.H. was impaired. The uppermost pictures represent a flag and a hammer. The words are "parents," "easy," and "giant." The lower pictures represent an anchor and a boat.

associative agnosia? Yes, although we must now admit that the distinction between apperceptive and associative agnosia is not the simple dichotomy originally proposed by Lissauer, of agnosia with and without impaired perception. Rather, the distinction is between agnosia with different kinds of visual impairments. Associative agnosics can draw or match visually presented objects that they cannot name, indicating far greater preservation of vision than is true of the apperceptive agnosics (in the narrow sense). Also unlike apperceptive agnosics, who guess at object identity based on color and texture cues, associative agnosics make use of shape information: When they err in object identification, it is often by naming an object that is similar in shape to the stimulus. Unlike dorsal simultanagnosics, associative agnosics have no difficulty detecting the presence of stimuli. The relation between ventral simultanagnosics and associative agnosics is somewhat less clear, in that at least some cases of associative agnosia show the same letter-by-letter reading impairment that characterizes ventral simultanagnosia. Nevertheless, the classic cases of ventral simultanagnosia described earlier are sufficiently preserved in their ability to carry out everyday object recognition that it seems appropriate to classify them separately, at least for now.

Notwithstanding these differences between the apperceptive agnosias and associative agnosia, it is clear that the perceptual capabilities of associative agnosics have been overstated by many authors. Empirically, the apperceptive-associative distinction does not seem to be a distinction between agnosia in which perception is "at fault" and agnosia in which it is not. In each case of associative agnosia in which higher levels of perception have been rigorously tested, they have been found to be severely impaired. Furthermore, although the nature of the perceptual abilities called upon by the different tests is not entirely clear, there does seem to be a certain "family resemblance" among them, involving the overall structure or configuration of a complex stimulus.

The neuropathology in these cases does not show great consistency, and attempted generalizations have themselves been varied: For example, Warrington (1985) states that associative agnosia has been described "most commonly in patients with diffuse cerebral disease. However, in those few well-documented cases in whom the lesion has been lateralized, the lateralization has been to the left hemisphere" (p. 342). In contrast, Alexander and Albert (1983) assert that the characteristic lesions are neither diffuse nor lateralized, but rather result from "bilateral damage to the inferior temporo-occipital junction" typically caused by strokes of the posterior cerebral artery distribution (p. 413).

Of the cases with localizing information, most can be described as having bilateral occipito-temporal damage. However, some cases appear to involve only unilateral damage to the occipital lobe and bordering posterior temporal or parietal lobe, on the left side in some cases (e.g., Boudouresques et al., 1972, case 1; Feinberg, Gonzalez-Rothi, and Heilman, 1986; Pillon, Signoret, and Lhermitte, 1981; Hecaen and Ajuriaguerra, 1956; and McCarthy and Warrington, 1986) and on the right side in others (e.g., Boudouresques, Poncet, Cherif, and Balzamo, 1979; and Levine, 1978).[2] The possibility that these different neuropathological settings for associative agnosia correspond to different perceptual impairments underlying associative agnosia will be explored in the next chapter.

Of the patients described above, the scope of the agnosic deficit varies somewhat from case to case. The dissociations among categories of stimuli that are and are not recognized by visual agnosics have been of interest to many writers because of the implications these dissociations have for the functional architecture of visual object recognition. Perhaps the most zealous use of this form of inference in the study of agnosia was made by Konorski (1967), who conjectured that there are nine different "gnostic fields" underlying human pattern recognition ability. He inferred a nine-part organization of the visual recognition system, shown in figure 20, based on a series of dissociations observed in individual patients. Although Konorski's observations are largely anecdotal, at least some of the distinctions embodied in his theory are supported by more widely observed and more thoroughly documented dissociations. For example, visual word recognition (reading) may be impaired or not in associative agnosia, as may face recognition. In some cases face recognition may seem to be the only aspect of visual object recognition that is impaired. Furthermore, recognition of facial identity may be impaired independent of recognition of facial emotion, and vice versa. Some patients seem to have more difficulty recognizing animate, or living, objects than inanimate objects. In the next section we will consider the different forms that selectively spared or impaired visual recognition can take.

4.2 Prosopagnosia

One of the most dramatic dissociations in neuropsychology is prosopagnosia, the inability to recognize faces despite intact intellectual functioning and even apparently intact visual recognition of most other stimuli. Bodamer introduced the term "prosopagnosia" in 1947, in conjunction with a careful study of three cases, and many cases have been reported in the neurological literature since then. A particularly complete description of a prosopagnosic patient is given by Pallis (1955):

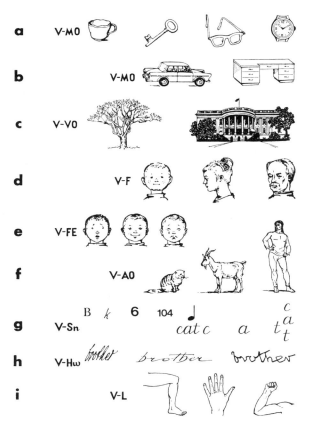

Figure 20
Konorski's nine different visual-gnostic categories, inferred on the basis of neuropsychological dissociations. (a) small, manipulable objects; (b) larger, partially manipulable objects; (c) nonmanipulable objects; (d) human faces; (e) emotional facial expressions; (f) animated objects; (g) signs; (h) handwriting; (i) positions of limbs.

He was of above average intelligence and his general level of awareness was extremely keen. His memory was remarkable... His span of digit retention was 8 forward and 6 backwards. There was no hesitation in his speech and he could obey complex orders. He read smoothly and there was no trouble in understanding and later describing what he had read . . . He promptly recognized, named, and demonstrated the use of a wide variety of test objects . . . The significance of line drawings was immediately apparent to him, and he could accurately describe the content of various pictures he was shown.

He mixed readily with the other patients on the ward, but rarely spoke unless spoken to first. He could not identify his medical attendants. "You must be a doctor because of your white coat, but I don't know which one you are. I'll know if you speak." He failed to identify his wife during visiting hours. She was told one day, without his possible knowledge, to walk right past his bed, but he did not show the least sign of recognition. Repeated attempts were made to 'catch him out' but none succeeded. If the disability was a feigned one, it was a performance of quite unbelievable virtuosity and consistency . . . He failed to identify pictures of Mr. Churchill, Mr. Aneurin Bevan, Hitler, Stalin, Miss Marilyn Monroe, or Mr. Groucho Marx. When confronted with such portraits he would proceed deductively, analyzing one feature after another, searching for the 'critical detail' which would yield the answer. In human faces, this was rarely forthcoming. There was somewhat less difficulty with animal faces. A goat was eventually recognized by its ears and beard, a giraffe by its neck, a crocodile by its dentition, and a cat by its whiskers . . .

The patient had analysed his difficulty in identifying faces with considerable insight. "I can see the eyes, nose, and mouth quite clearly, but they just don't add up. They all seem chalked in, like on a blackboard . . . I have to tell by the clothes or by the voice whether it is a man or a woman . . . The hair may help a lot, or if there is a mustache . . .

"At the club I saw someone strange staring at me, and asked the steward who it was. You'll laugh at me. I'd been looking at myself in a mirror."

Many other cases of profound impairment in face recognition, with little or no agnosia for other stimuli, have been reported in the literature, including Assal, Favre, and Anderes (1984); Bornstein and Kidron (1959); Cole and Perez-Cruet (1964); De Renzi (1986); Kay and Levin (1982); Lhermitte and Pillon (1975); Nardelli, Buonanno, Coccia, Fiaschi, Terzian, and Rizzuto, (1982); Shuttleworth, Syring, and Allen (1982); and Whitely and Warrington (1977). Other cases are listed in table 1 of the next chapter.

How selective is the recognition impairment in prosopagnosia? There are different dimensions along which one can measure selectivity. For example, within the realm of face recognition, one can ask whether the impairment in the recognition of facial identity is dissociated from impairments in the recognition of facial expression. Although the recognition of facial expression is not always tested in cases of prosopagnosia, and when it is it is sometimes found to be impaired, there are cases in which the recognition of facial expression is preserved (e.g., Bruyer et al., 1983; Shuttleworth, Syring, and Allen, 1982, case 2). In Bruyer et al.'s case, for example, the patient was unable to recognize photographs of famous faces or videotapes of himself, his family, and his physicians. Nevertheless, he was able to match photographs of different faces according to whether they had the same facial expression and judge the appropriateness of different facial expressions evoked by stimuli such as a clown or a funeral. The possibility that this dissociation might result from emotion being an easier facial characteristic to recognize than identity is allayed by the finding of the opposite pattern of dissociation in other patients: Kurucz and Feldmar (1979) found that certain patients classified as having "chronic organic brain syndrome" were able to recognize photographs of famous faces and yet were unable to identify facial expressions of either drawn or photographed faces.

Etcoff (1984) has directly tested the hypothesis that the visual recognition of facial identity and facial expression are subserved by distinct "modules," using a sorting task in which photographs of faces must be put in separate piles depending upon either their identity or their expression. The speed and accuracy with which normal subjects perform this task is not affected by whether facial identity is correlated with facial expression (i.e., a certain person always has a certain expression), implying that normal subjects process these two properties of faces independently: That is, they can just recognize identity without automatically recognizing expression, and vice versa. Right-, but not left-, hemisphere-damaged patients differed from normal subjects in this task in that their sorting performance was influenced by the irrelevant dimension, as if their specialized modules for recognizing identity independent of expression and expression independent of identity were damaged. Etcoff's conclusion that two separate modules underlie the recognition of facial identity and facial expression, but that they are neuroanatomical neighbors, is consistent with the case report literature, showing some degree of association between the two abilities with occasional dissociations.

The selectivity of prosopagnosia can also be assessed in terms of the range of types of stimuli that patients are no longer able to recognize. Although an impairment in face recognition is by definition the most prominent deficit in prosopagnosia, many of these patients have difficulty recognizing other types of stimuli as well. For example, it has already been mentioned that Pallis's patient had difficulty recognizing animal faces. Difficulty recognizing animals (faces or whole bodies) is often present in prosopagnosia. In some cases, this problem is confined to the recognition of animals within a class. For example, Bornstein's (1963) case was a birdwatcher who could no longer distinguish among different species, saying, "All the birds look the same" (p. 284), and the patient described in a brief report by Newcombe (1979) was reported to have lost the ability to individuate racehorses. The patient described by Bornstein, Sroka, and Munitz (1969) was a farmer who had previously been able to distinguish his cows individually, but lost this ability when he became prosopagnosic. A similar case was described by Assal, Favre, and Anderes (1984) under the syndrome name 'zooagnosia'. This case has drawn particular attention because the patient's prosopagnosia improved while the impairment in recognizing individual cows remained. Although this has been cited as evidence that animal recognition impairments are separable from human face recognition impairments (e.g., Young, 1988), it should be borne in mind that the task of recognizing individual cows is probably more difficult than the task of recognizing individual humans, and that the Assal et al. case did remain mildly prosopagnosic: After his "recovery" from prosopagnosia, he would sometimes hesitate in identifying people and occasionally make an error (p. 581).

In addition to within-species distinctions, many prosopagnosic patients have also been reported to have trouble distinguishing between animals of different species. For example, Shuttleworth, Syring, and Allen's (1982) case 2 was able to recognize only two out of twelve color photographs of common animals, making flagrant errors, such as calling geese "fish" because of the surrounding water. The patients studied by Boudouresques et al. (1979); Damasio, Damasio, and VanHoesen (1982); Gomori and Hawryluk (1984); Lhermitte, Chain, Escourelle, Ducarne, and Pillon (1972); Lhermitte and Pillon (1975), and Pallis (1955) all showed similar problems of varying degree in recognizing the species depicted in animal pictures.

It might not seem surprising that damage to the mechanisms underlying face recognition would be accompanied by impairments in recognizing individual animals, or even the general species of animals. What is more unexpected is the finding that prosopagnosics have been noted to have specific problems recognizing plants (Boudouresques et al., 1979;

Gomori and Hawryluk, 1984; Whitely and Warrington, 1977, case 1) and even man-made stimuli such as buildings and public monuments (Assal et al., 1984; Bornstein and Kidron, 1959; Boudouresques et al., 1979; Gomori and Hawryluk, 1984; Lhermitte, et al. 1972; Lhermitte and Pillon, 1975; Pallis, 1955; Shuttleworth et al., 1982, case 2), makes of automobile (Boudouresques et al., 1979; Damasio, et al., 1982; Gomori and Hawryluk, 1984; Lhermitte et al., 1972; Lhermitte and Pillon, 1975; Newcombe, 1979; Shuttleworth et al., 1982, case 2), and articles of clothing (Damasio et al., 1982; Shuttleworth et al., 1982, case 2). Food is another category of stimuli with which prosopagnosics may experience difficulty (Damasio et al., 1982; Michel et al., 1986; Whitely and Warrington, 1977). For example, the case of Michel et al. had so much trouble recognizing food that she resorted to organizing her refrigerator in a special way, with each type of food assigned a fixed location. Similarly, Damasio et al.'s case 1 "would confuse foodstuffs and required help in her cooking. To select articles from the shelves of the supermarket, she had to read every label, whereas before, the mere shape and size of containers would permit the correct choice" (p. 338).

It is difficult to know whether impairments in recognizing these nonface stimuli are common in prosopagnosia, or whether the cases cited above constitute a special group. Although many published case reports on prosopagnosia do not mention impairments in visual recognition outside of human faces, this does not necessarily mean that recognition of animals, buildings, and so on was carefully tested and found to be normal in these cases. Even when the authors report that they tested recognition of nonface stimuli and found it to be normal, some caution should be exercised in interpreting these results. The recognition of objects other than faces tends to be treated as a rather peripheral topic in many reports of prosopagnosia and is therefore often examined and described rather cursorily. For example, the patient of Cole and Perez-Cruet (1964) was described in their case report as not having object agnosia, and yet the authors also report that "there was a definite rise in the temporal threshold for recognition [of pictures and words] as measured tachistoscopically at times in the range of 1, 5, 10 or even 15 seconds" and add that some pictures of objects were not recognized even with unlimited viewing time (p. 240)!

The most compelling evidence for preserved recognition of stimuli other than faces was reported by De Renzi (1986). His case 4 was sufficiently prosopagnosic that "the identification of relatives and close friends constituted an insurmountable problem if he could not rely upon their voices" (p. 246). Nevertheless, he was able to distinguish among subtly different objects: "He was requested to identify his own electric razor, wallet, glasses, and neckties when each of them was presented together with six to ten objects of the same category, chosen as to have physical resemblance with the target. He was also asked to write a sentence on a cardboard and then to identify his own handwriting from nine samples of the same sentence written by other persons. Finally, he was required to identify the photograph of a Siamese cat from photographs of other cats and to sort out 20 Italian coins from 20 foreign coins. On all of these tasks he performed unhesitatingly and correctly. It must be added that on inquiry both the patient and his wife denied that he had ever shown any problem in the identification of personal objects. He easily recognized his car in parking lots" (p. 249). Although other tests, including tachistoscopic stimulus presentations, might have shown *some* impairment in the recognition of nonface objects, De Renzi's data provide at least a lower bound on how selective face recognition impairments can be, and they do demonstrate an impressively large degree of selectivity.

Yet another dimension of selectivity that has been investigated in prosopagnosia is the extent to which the recognition impairment is dissociable from perceptual impairments. As with the more general category of associative agnosia, there is some controversy over just how intact the visual perception of prosopagnosics is. The most frequently cited test of perception in prosopagnosics is Benton and Van Allen's (1968) matching task. This task consists of a series of photographs of unfamiliar faces, viewed from the front, each of which must be matched with one of a set of six other photographs. Some of these sets of six photographs have been taken from a different angle or under different lighting conditions. An example is shown in figure 21. How do prosopagnosics perform on this task? There is a range of performance across different cases, and different authors focus on different portions of this range. For example, Damasio (1985) cites the research of Benton and Van Allen (e.g., 1972; Benton, 1980) in support of the claim that these patients' "perception of both the whole and the parts of a facial stimulus is intact . . . Prosopagnosic patients are generally able to perform complex perceptual tasks (such as the Benton and Van Allen test of unfamiliar facial discrimination)" (p. 263). Benton and Van Allen's (1972) statement is somewhat less strong: "The disabilities underlying prosopagnosia and impairment in performance on the visuoperceptive task of discriminating unfamiliar faces are, or at least may be, dissociable" (p. 170). This conclusion was based on a review of three cases of prosopagnosia, one of which was "markedly impaired" at discriminating faces and two of which were "essentially normal" (p. 168), as well a new case, who performed "on a mediocre level, but within broad normal limits" (p. 169) on their test of face discrimination.

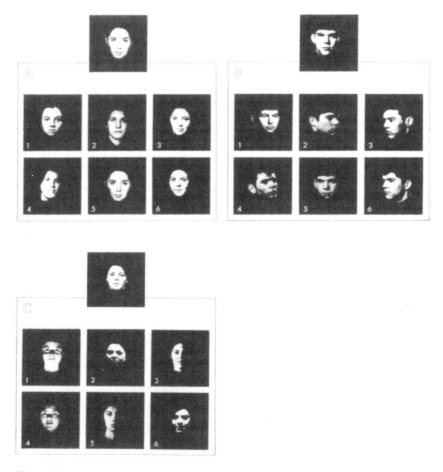

Figure 21
Sample items from Benton and Van Allen's Test of Facial Recognition. In part A the subject is required to match identical front views of faces. In part B the subject is required to match faces across changes in viewing angle. In part C the subject is required to match faces across changes in lighting.

In contrast, Shuttleworth, Syring, and Allen (1982) conclude that face discrimination deficits are closely associated with prosopagnosia. They reviewed the English language literature for cases of prosopagnosia and found approximately 100 cases, 18 of which were described in considerable detail. Their summary of the face discrimination capabilities of these patients is as follows: "Of the four cases in which matching of identical face photographs [which can be accomplished though serial feature by feature matching] was specifically reported, all were unimpaired except for slowness of performance. In contrast, matching of nonidentical poses was found to be abnormal in mild to definite degree in 12 of 13 patients in whom this task was reported . . . Even from briefly described cases it was apparent that most patients had subjective visual complaints (approximately 85 percent of 44 cases) usually described as blurring or loss of color, and some degree of metamorphosia [distortion of faces] was common, being noted in approximately 60–65 percent of cases" (p. 313). Shuttleworth et al.'s observation that a global memory disorder was present in 17 of 46 prosopagnosics (p. 318) must also be taken into account in evaluating dissociations between the recognition of previously familiar faces and the discrimination of unfamiliar faces. For example, Malone, Morris, Kay, and Levin's (1982) report of a prosopagnosic, which was published too late to be included in Shuttleworth et al.'s literature review, has been cited as "the strongest evidence" for impaired face recognition with roughly intact face discrimination (Young, 1987). This patient had memory impairments and was initially impaired at face discrimination, although he later performed in the "average range" (no score or time given). It is therefore conceivable that his face recognition deficit resulted from the combined effects of a modality-general memory impairment and low-normal ability to perceive faces.

A further uncertainty related to the interpretation of preserved face discrimination performance in cases of prosopagnosia has been pointed out by Newcombe (1979). She observed a prosopagnosic patient who performed well on tests of face matching and discrimination, but required lengthy inspections of the faces, and, by his own report, relied on specific local features such as the shape of the hairline. When the faces were shown to him with oval frames blocking the hairline, his performance dropped markedly. Newcombe points out that "Some prosopagnosic patients are reported to match faces normally . . . Latencies, however, are not invariably measured. Where they are, they are described as abnormally slow" (p. 319). This tells us that the final score of patients could be within normal limits when in fact their ability to perceive faces is clearly abnormal.

What about the other half of the double dissociation between face discrimination performance and face recognition? The existence of nonprosopagnosic patients who perform poorly on face discrimination tasks would appear to strengthen the hypothesis that prosopagnosia is not invariably associated with impairments in face perception, insofar as it shows that the visual discrimination deficit is not alone sufficient to cause prosopagnosia (e.g., Benton, 1980; Damasio, 1985). However, just as prosopagnosic patients may succeed at face discrimination tasks for reasons different from those of normal subjects (i.e., through laborious feature by feature comparison), nonprosopagnosic patients may fail face discrimination tasks for different reasons than prosopagnosic patients fail. The observation that nonprosopagnosic patients may perform poorly on these face discrimination tasks than prosopagnosic patients is only relevant if we assume that the two groups of patients find the discrimination tasks difficult *for the same reasons.* To take a very simple example, visual neglect will cause a patient to perform poorly on the discrimination test because he will neglect some of the multiple choice alternatives (see figure 21). Thus, poor performance on this test need not be the result of a specific inability to construct visual face representations. Without knowing what aspects of the discrimination test are found difficult by prosopagnosic and nonprosopagnosic patients, the finding that nonprosopagnosic patients may do worse than prosopagnosic patients on the face discrimination test cannot be definitively interpreted.

A group study of unilaterally brain-damaged patients by Warrington and James (1967) is often cited as evidence for the independence of deficits in face recognition and face discrimination, with the implication that a face recognition deficit could occur independently of a face discrimination deficit in prosopagnosia. In this research, left- and right-hemisphere-damaged patients and control subjects were given two tests: A famous faces recognition test in which photos of well-known politicians and actors were to be identified, and an unfamiliar face discrimination test, in which a photo of an unfamiliar face was shown for ten seconds, followed immediately by eight photos of faces from which the subject was to select the one just shown. Warrington and James report that right-hemisphere-damaged patients as a group performed worse on both tests, but that there was no relation between their performance on the two tests, implying that the tests tap different abilities. However, lack of a significant relation is a null result of sorts, and several considerations argue that in this case it may be due to insufficient sensitivity of the research design and data analysis. The first such consideration is the small number of items in each test: ten in the famous faces and eight in the unfamiliar faces. The second is the generally low rate of errors on these tests, approaching a ceiling effect: The right-hemisphere- damaged patients, who performed the worst, made an average of only two errors on the famous faces test and one and a half on the unfamiliar faces test. (Note that chance performance is effectively zero on the first test and .125 on the second.) Finally, the test of the strength of relationship between the two tests within the right-hemisphere-damaged group was weak: Patients were divided into two categories for each test, depending upon whether they made more or less than two errors on each test, and the strength of relationship between the two tests was carried out on the sheer number of patients above and below the cut off for each test.

To summarize, most prosopagnosics have impaired visual perception of faces, as measured by their ability to discriminate between photographs of unfamiliar faces, and even those cases with reportedly preserved face discrimination ability may be using special strategies. Of course, lack of firm evidence for prosopagnosia with intact face perception is not the same as firm evidence for a lack of prosopagnosia with intact face perception. Such cases may exist, and future reports may document them appropriately, including information about the strategies used by the patients in performing the face discrimination tasks. Nevertheless, the current evidence suggests that prosopagnosics do not *perceive* faces normally.

In addition to delineating the prosopagnosic deficit in terms of its selectivity for recognition of facial identity versus facial expression, recognition of faces versus other objects, and recognition of faces versus "mere" perception of faces, it may be possible in some cases to separate impaired awareness of recognition from impaired recognition. Several recent investigations of prosopagnosic patients have revealed evidence of face recognition in tasks that test recognition implicitly, that is, without requiring the subject to make a conscious decision about the familiarity or identity of the face. There are two general ways in which this has been accomplished. One approach has been to use psychophysiological measures of subjects' responses to faces, including skin conductance responses (SCRs) and event-related brain potentials (ERPs). For example, Bauer (1984) presented a prosopagnosic patient with a series of photographs of familiar faces. While viewing each face, the patient heard a list of names read aloud, one of which was the name of the person in the photograph. For normal subjects in this paradigm (originally developed by forensic psychologists and known as the "guilty knowledge" test), SCR to a name is greater when the named face is shown than when a different face is shown. Although the prosopagnosic's SCR to the names was not as strongly correlated with the photographs as normal subjects', it was nevertheless significantly correlated. In contrast, the patient performed at chance levels when asked to select the correct name for each face. Tranel and Damasio (1985) showed that a prosopagnosic patient had generally larger SCRs to familiar than unfamiliar faces, even though she rated all of the faces as unfamiliar. More recent studies have reached similar conclusions using ERPs (Renault, Signoret, Debruille, Breton and Bolgert, 1989), and have demonstrated that familiarity effects are present only for previously familiar faces and not those presented earlier in a testing session (Bauer and Verfaellie, 1988).

Another set of studies has converged on the same conclusions using conventional behavioral measures such as reaction time or trials to learning criterion in tasks involving face stimuli. For example, de Haan, Young and Newcombe (1987) found that, like normal subjects, a prosopagnosic patient was faster at classifying the printed names of famous people as politicians or not if a simultaneously presented face was from the same category (e.g., the face of a politician if the name was of a politician) and slower if the face was from the other category (e.g., the face of a politician if the name was of a nonpolitician). Bruyer, Laterre, Seron, Feyereisen, Strypstein, Pierrard, and Rectem (1983) showed that a prosopagnosic patient was able to learn pairings of famous names and famous faces faster if the pairings were correct than if they were incorrect, a finding replicated by De Haan et al. (1987) with their case. However, Newcombe, Young and De Haan (1989) failed to observe this savings in learning time for another case, and concluded that covert recognition is not invariably present in prosopagnosia.

Claims of cognition without awareness in cognitive psychology and neuropsychology have rightfully been met with some degree of skepticism. The history of such topics as subliminal reading in normal subjects (e.g., Holender, 1986; Marcel, 1983) or blindsight in cortically blind subjects (e.g., Campion, Latto and Smith, 1983; Weiskrantz, 1986) has revealed the many methodological pitfalls and conceptual difficulties that beset any attempt to empirically separate cognition and awareness of cognition, and expert opinion is still divided on these issues. Research on covert recognition in prosopagnosia shares many of the same problems. For example, it has so far been impossible to equate measures of covert recognition in prosopagnosics and in normal subjects, because prosopagnosics' SCRs are weaker, their reaction times are longer, and so forth. Therefore, the most that can be said is that they have some degree of covert recognition, and not that they have normal recognition when tested covertly. This raises the possibility that the covert measures are just more sensitive measures of the same recognition processes tested overtly, and are not indexing a true dissociation between conscious and unconscious recognition. Whether there is such a dissociation can only be settled by a careful assessment of the overt recognition ability of these patients as well as their covert recognition performance, and by a thorough understanding of the relation between covert and overt measures in general (i.e., how they scale against each other in normal subjects and whether moderately impaired performance on overt measures is normally associated with performance towards the high end of the range on covert measures). Unfortunately, little attention has been paid to these issues. For example, De Haan et al. refer to their patient as performing "at chance" in an overt test of the politician/nonpolitician face judgement task, but in fact his 30 correct answers out of 48 trials has only a .06 probability of being the product of random guessing, suggesting some residual overt face recognition ability. The uniform "unfamiliar" responses of Tranel and Damasio's case to the photographed faces used in their experiments could reflect a complete inability to recognize consciously the familiar faces, or it could reflect an only partial impairment in conscious recognition paired with a conservative response bias. Whether these kinds of problems should be considered minor methodological imperfections or important sources of artifact is difficult to know at present.

The neuropathology of prosopagnosia has received much attention. All writers agree that a right hemisphere lesion is necessary. Discussion has focussed on the intrahemispheric location of the right hemisphere lesion and the necessity for a second, left hemisphere lesion. Benton and Van Allen (1972) suggest that the critical lesion site for prosopagnosia may be in the "parieto-occipital area of the right hemisphere (or perhaps of both hemispheres)" (p. 171). Meadows (1974) reviewed the clinical case literature on prosopagnosia, using visual field defects and autopsy reports to infer the distribution of lesion sites. The almost invariable finding of a left superior quadrananopia implicates the right *inferior* anterior occipital, or occipito*temporal*, region in prosopagnosia, and this conclusion was supported by the findings in those cases that came to autopsy. In addition, autopsy data indicated that a second, sometimes smaller, lesion was always present in the homologous regions of the left hemisphere. Although more recently some authors have reported cases of prosopagnosia following unilateral right posterior (usually inferior occipitotemporal) damage (De Renzi, 1986; Landis, Cummings, Christen, Bogen, and Imhof, 1986; Whitely and Warrington, 1977), none of these cases has come to autopsy, raising the possibility of left hemisphere dysfunction not apparent from clinical and radiological information. This possibility is made more likely by the recent reports of additional autopsied cases with bilateral lesions. Nardelli, Buonanno, Coccia, Fiaschi, Terzian, and Rizzuto (1982) describe four cases of prosopagnosia, one of which had pathological verification and showed bilateral inferior occipitotemporal lesions. Damasio, Damasio, and Van Hoesen (1982) and Damasio (1985) present additional evidence favoring a ventral, rather than dorsal, localization for prosopagnosia, and also confirming the necessity for bilateral, symmetrical lesions. Calling upon data from both autopsy and brain imaging techniques (CT, MRI, SPECT), Damasio and associates argue that the inferior occipitotemporal regions of the brain must be damaged bilaterally to produce prosopagnosia.

4.3 Pure Alexia

Patients with pure alexia cannot read normally, despite visual capabilities that appear normal on informal testing, and despite their ability to understand spoken language and to write. Their alexia is called "pure" because of the preservation of writing and other language-related abilities, which leads to the almost paradoxical phenomenon of these patients' inability to read something that they themselves have just written. Typically, they read words letter by letter, spelling each word before identifying it. Even when they do not spell aloud, analysis of their single word reading latencies, as a function of number of letters in the word, suggests a letter-by-letter strategy. Figure 22 shows the monotonic, almost perfectly linear, dependence of reading latency on word length in a pure alexic patient studied by Bub, Black, and Howell (1989). The negative acceleration of this function is probably attributable to the greater possibility of guessing the word before the last letters are read

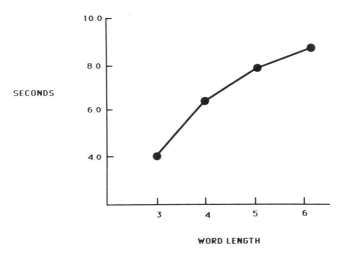

Figure 22
Single word reading latency as a function of number of letters in the word for a pure alexic patient studied by Bub et al. (1989).

with longer words. Note the time scale on this figure: Even short words require several seconds for this patient, and each additional letter adds a second or more to the reading time. In a review of cases of pure alexia for which single word reading latencies were recorded, Shallice (1988, chapter 4) found that the time needed to read three- to four-letter words ranged from just under 2 seconds to 17 seconds, and the time needed for seven- to eight-letter words ranged from 3 seconds to almost 47 seconds. In these same cases, the percentage of individual letters within a word read correctly ranged from 100 percent to only 50 percent. Shallice points out that in most cases letters are read more accurately than words, although letters are rarely read perfectly.

Pure alexia has often been viewed as a category-specific visual agnosia. For example, in his textbook on behavioral neurology, Mesulam (1985) states that "pure alexia is essentially a visual agnosia for verbal material" (p. 18). This is a reasonable view, given the apparent selectivity of the impairment for just verbal material in the visual modality. In addition, many, although not all, cases of associative agnosia also suffer from pure alexia, strengthening the notion that pure alexia is a form of visual associative agnosia.

In contrast to associative object agnosia and prosopagnosia, which we know about mainly through descriptive case reports, most of the available data on pure alexia have been collected within the context of experimental investigations. The main objective of these investigations has been to arrive at a proper interpretation of the syndrome, in terms of the components of normal processing that have been impaired. Therefore, a more detailed presentation of the empirical findings on pure alexia will be deferred until the next chapter, when theoretical interpretations for the associative agnosic syndromes are discussed.

4.4 Other Categories

4.4.1 Living and nonliving things

Warrington and her colleagues have described a set of individual cases in which knowledge of stimuli roughly corresponding to "living things" is relatively impaired compared to knowledge of most "nonliving things," or in which knowledge of "nonliving things" is relatively impaired compared to that of "living things." "Living things" appear to comprise animals, plants, and foods; "nonliving things" are most typically exemplified by small, manipulable, man-made objects. The patients who show selective deficits for either of these broad categories do not appear to be visual associative agnosics in the sense of having a selective deficit in visual recognition. Indeed, their impairments are, if anything, more apparent in purely verbal tasks, such as naming the word corresponding to a spoken definition. However, in several, but not all, of the cases, the impairment cannot be attributed soley to verbal processes, as it is evident even in tasks that do not stress language: Miming the use of objects (Warrington and Shallice, 1984), describing the object in lieu of naming it (Warrington and Shallice, 1984), and sorting visually dissimilar but semantically related pictures (Warrington and McCarthy, 1987). In terms of Warrington's framework for object recognition, shown in figure 15, these patients are interpreted as having impaired "semantic categorization," and Warrington refers to them as associative agnosics. A useful overview and synthesis of the literature on these cases and other neuropsychological evidence concerning semantics may be found in Shallice (1988, chapter 12).

4.4.2 Super-selective category-specific impairments
In recent years a number of highly specific deficits in the processing of particular categories of stimuli have been reported to follow brain damage. These include deficits confined to body parts (Dennis, 1976), objects typically found indoors (Yamadori and Albert, 1973), and fruits and vegetables (Hart, Berndt, and Caramazza, 1985). Although most discussions of these phenomena have understandably focussed on the striking specificity of the impairments, an equally important question is: Which cognitive or perceptual systems have been impaired? For present purposes, the important issue is whether or not they reflect an underlying deficit in *visual recognition*, or whether they involve impairments in other cognitive processes required for naming visually presented objects.

   So far, the results of testing these patients on a variety of visual and verbal tasks indicates that the locus of impairment is linguistic. For example, the intriguing case M.D. of Hart, Berndt and Caramazza (1985) was unable to name fruits and vegetables as common as oranges or peaches, although he could quickly supply the names of such unusual items as an abacus or a sphinx. Hart et al. charted the boundaries of M.D.'s impairment in a variety of tasks, including visual and auditory lexical decision, oral reading, word-picture matching, semantic categorization of pictures and words, and picture naming. The results of this exhaustive testing were fairly clear: M.D. was unable to access the names of *just* fruits and vegetables, and this was true whether he was naming a visually or tactilely presented stimulus or naming from a verbal definition. In contrast, he had no trouble understanding the names of these items. Most relevant to the present concerns, he had no trouble recognizing fruits and vegetables, as evidenced by perfect performance on a picture-word matching task.³ Similarly, in the other cases of superselective category-specific impairment, the locus of impairment seems to be confined to lexical operations and does not affect visual recognition per se.

4.4.3 Relation between associative visual object agnosia and narrower categorical recognition deficits

On the face of things, the deficits in knowledge of "living" and "nonliving" things seem distinct from visual agnosia, in that these patients do not invariably have visual recognition deficits (e.g., Warrington and McCarthy, 1983), and when they do have recognition impairments they are part of a more pervasive loss of knowledge, at least as evident in purely verbal tasks as in visual tasks. Therefore, for purposes of an initial taxonomy, these patients seem to belong in a separate category from the visual agnosics whose deficits seem confined to visual recognition per se. Similarly, the superselective category-specific deficits just described appear to result from impairments outside of the visual recognition system, as they are confined to lexical/semantic operations. It seems that they, too, comprise a distinct class of neuropsychological phenomena from the visual agnosias.

In contrast, there seems to be no clear dividing line between prosopagnosia and the across-the-board associative object agnosias reviewed earlier. Indeed, many cases have been cited by one author as a case of object agnosia and by another as a case of prosopagnosia. Given that the recognition impairment in prosopagnosia often extends beyond human faces, there is no obvious discontinuity between prosopagnosia and object agnosia. The line between pure alexia and object agnosia is not much clearer, particularly in view of the following two facts: that the recognition deficit in at least some cases of pure alexia is not confined to verbal material (e.g., Kinsbourne and Warrington, 1962), and that some cases of pure alexia are impaired at recognizing even single forms.

4.5 Optic Aphasia

There are patients with visual modality-specific naming disorders, called optic aphasia, who cannot name visually presented objects. The distinction between these patients and the associative agnosics discussed earlier has not always been made clearly in the literature, and there is disagreement over the relation between the two syndromes. Some authors have theorized that associative agnosia is nothing but optic aphasia (Geschwind, 1965). Others have assumed a less extreme, but also less clear, position, stating that optic aphasia is equivalent to a *mild* associative agnosia (e.g., Bauer and Rubens, 1985; Kertesz, 1987). Still others have suggested that optic aphasia is a *type* of associative agnosia, in which perception is truly normal (Humphreys and Riddoch, 1987). On the face of things, patients with optic aphasia do not appear to have agnosia, as they can indicate their recognition of objects nonverbally, even when they cannot name them. In addition, their condition cannot be attributed to a general anomia, as they can provide the correct word when given an auditorily presented sentence frame or a definition.

The abilities and impairments of patients with optic aphasia have posed a serious challenge to cognitive neuropsychological explanation. Conventional models of the functional architecture underlying visual naming, which include visual structural descriptions, "semantics" (either modality-general or modality-specific) and various language operations, do not easily accomodate these patients. Because of the close association in the literature between optic aphasia and associative agnosia, and also because of the implications for the functional architecture underyling visual naming, these patients will be described in some detail here.

One of the most thoroughly studied cases of optic aphasia was described by Lhermitte and Beauvois (1973). Their subject, Jules F., suffered a posterior left hemisphere stroke, with some amnesia, pure alexia, and mild constructional apraxia and color vision deficit. Although he made relatively few errors in naming objects from verbal definition (5/125), or from their characteristic noises or their feel in his hand (1/25 and 11/120, respectively), he made a large number of errors (35/130) in naming visually presented objects and pictures. Although he performed well on a task of pointing to a visual stimulus depicting a spoken name, the authors point out that the choice set of possible responses in this task is much smaller than in the naming tasks just described, suggesting that performance in this task may not be truly better than in naming visually presented stimuli when overall difficulty is accounted for. They also point out that when the named item was absent, Jules pointed to incorrect choices that were semantically related to the word, apparently without any awareness that the correct choice was missing.

Based on his naming performance in different modalities, it is clear that Jules F. is not simply anomic, but has a specific problem naming visual stimuli. However, the data so far are consistent with his being a visual agnosic, or even blind. The second critical element for classifying him as an optic aphasic is the ability to demonstrate recognition of visually presented stimuli by means other than naming. A common nonverbal means of communicating recognition, often used spontaneously by patients like Jules F., is to gesture the use of the object in pantomime. Lhermitte and Beauvois presented the patient with 100 pictures of common objects, and report that whenever he mimed the use of an object he did so correctly, even when he misnamed the object. For example, when shown a picture of a boot, he mimed pulling on a boot but called it a hat. Thus, the authors conclude that the visual naming deficit cannot be attributed to agnosia. Consistent with this is their observation that the patient had no trouble interacting with the visual world in everyday life. They do mention occasional agnosialike behavior with certain complex objects: He can sometimes copy or describe the appearance of a stimulus accurately without being able to identify it by any means.

The patient's errors in naming visual stimuli seemed to be mainly semantic in nature, with many perseverations of responses from previous trials. Visual errors without semantic similarity were reported to be relatively rare, although many errors showed both visual and semantic similarity to the correct response. When given unlimited time to name a visual stimulus, Jules F. would generally home in on the correct name. However, several attempts were often necessary, as is evident in the following protocol (Lhermitte and Beauvois, 1973, pp. 706–707):

> A grasshopper: "a cricket, not a cricket, a grasshopper."
> A mussel: "it looks like 2 snails, 2 slugs, it is a shellfish, not an oyster, it should be mussels then."
> A bus: "a wagon . . . a public transport since there is a back door . . . a stage-coach . . . it would be . . . no . . . a city cab .. . not a cab but a city bus."
> A window-blind: "A parasol, metallic curtain rods . . . the cloth roof . . . surrounding sails . . . it could be a parasol . . . there are rods, but isn't it a shelter? A window-blind."
> An aquarium: "A bird cage, unless it is a pot for flowers, a container, a tank, the four aspects . . . the walls made of glass or wood . . . it could be an aquarium if it is made of glass."
> A medieval crown: [a preceding picture had correctly been named "basket"] "a kind of foot of metallic basket, a basket for flowers, a basket for a table . . . it cannot be a basket for decoration on a table . . . it is not a decoration, I do not know what it could be . . . A basket with 4 feet, no with 4 crossed hoops . . . it cannot be worn as clothing, it would be a hat. It would be a very fancy hat to look like that . . ."

In order to determine whether objects were misnamed because they were misperceived, or whether the naming errors were generated after an adequate perceptual analysis was complete, Lhermitte and Beauvois asked the subject to draw what he had seen and what he had named on trials in which objects were misnamed. When asked to draw what he had seen, he invariably drew a recognizable picture of the stimulus, which was distinguishable from his drawing of the named item. For example, on one trial the stimulus was a tree and Jules F. said, "it's a house with a straw roof," a perseveration from a previous trial in which a house was shown. When requested to draw what he had seen, he drew a tree, insisting all the while that he was drawing a "straw roof." and when requested to draw a house, he produced a good drawing of a house. Lhermitte and Beauvois conclude that processing within the visual system is roughly intact and cannot be the cause of the errors in visual naming. Another observation that is consistent with this conclusion comes from testing with tachistoscopic stimulus presentations. Jules F. would often continue to search for and home in on the correct name for a picture long after the picture had disappeared, as if he had gotten sufficient visual information in the brief presentation and the laborious part of the visual naming process was postvisual.

A small number of other cases of optic aphasia have been described in the literature, including: Assal and Regli (1980); Coslett and Saffran (1989); Gil, Pluchon, Toullat, Micheneau, Rogez, and Lefevre (1985); Larrabee, et al. (case 2, 1985); Poeck, 1984; Riddoch and Humphreys (1987b); and Spreen, Benton, and Van Allen (1966). These cases show a strong similarity to that of Lhermitte and Beauvois in several respects: Naming is normal or relatively unimpaired for objects presented in the tactile modality (Assal and Regli, 1980; Coslett and Saffran, 1989; Larrabee et al., 1985; Poeck, 1984; Riddoch and Humphreys, 1987b; Spreen, Benton, and Van Allen, 1966) and for sounds (Assal and Regli, 1980; Gil et al., 1985; Spreen, Benton, and Van Allen, 1966), as well as to spoken definition (all cases). Reading, as well as naming of visually presented objects and pictures, is invariably performed poorly. Like the case of Lhermitte and Beauvois, two of these patients can demonstrate their recognition by gesturing appropriately to a visual stimulus (Gil et al., 1985; Riddoch and Humphreys, 1987b). In two other cases, the patients could not be discouraged from naming the objects before making their gestures, and the gestures would then be made for the named object rather than for the visually presented object (Coslett and Saffran, 1989; Larrabee et al, 1985). The patient described by Assal and Regli (1980) was as impaired at gesturing to visually presented stimuli as she was at naming them, and neither Poeck (1984) nor Spreen, Benton, and Van Allen (1980) report on gesturing in their cases.

With the exception of Spreen, Benton, and Van Allen (1980), who do not report the nature of the naming errors, all reports describe frequent semantic errors. For example, "vines" for a trellis (Coslett and Saffran, 1989), "cigarette lighter" for lamp (Gil et al., 1985), "bracelet" for necklace

(Poeck, 1984), and "toy car" for toy gun (Riddoch and Humpreys, 1987b). In all cases, perseverations were common. In two cases a large proportion of naming errors were reported to be completely unrelated to the visual stimulus (Assal and Regli, 1980; Coslett and Saffran, 1989), whereas in four others such errors were in a minority (Gil et al., 1985; Larrabee et al., 1985; Lhermitte and Beauvois, 1973; Riddoch and Humpreys, 1987).

Visual errors bearing no semantic relationship to the stimulus were relatively rare in these cases, although they were noted to occur occasionally in many cases (Coslett and Saffran, 1989; Gil et al., 1985; Lhermitte and Beauvois, 1973; Riddoch and Humpreys, 1987b). The visual quality of the stimulus has little or no effect on these patients' naming performance: When reported separately, the naming of objects, photographs, and drawings shows little or no difference (Gil et al., 1985; Larrabee et al., 1985; Lhermitte and Beauvois, 1973; Poeck, 1984; Riddoch and Humphreys, 1987b). Some of the more recent studies of optic aphasia have described nonverbal tests of visual recognition other than gesturing. One such test is an "object decision" task, in which the subject must distinguish between drawings of real objects and drawings of nonexistent objects, made by recombining parts of real objects. The ability to perform such a test implies that perception is adequate for recognition, and that visual memory contains representations of the depicted objects. The cases of Assal and Regli (1980), Riddoch and Humphreys (1987), and Coslett and Saffran (1989) all performed well on this type of task.

A variety of categorization tasks has been used to assess visual recognition in these cases. The most frequently used task requires the subject to sort together items from the same superordinate category, or items serving the same function. For example, given a set of pictures of furniture, vehicles, and animals, the subject is to put the items in the same categories together. All of the patients tested on such tasks did well on them, although performance was never perfect (Assal and Regli, 1980; Coslett and Saffran, 1989; Riddoch and Humphreys, 1987). Oddly, a very similar task designed by Riddoch and Humphreys proved extremely difficult for their subject. In this task, triads are presented, with the instruction to group together the two that are "associated with one another or would be used together," and set apart the third, which "might be from the same general class, but is either not associated with the target objects or is not used in conjunction with them." Examples of these triads are: cup, saucer, colander; candle, candleholder, light bulb; pencil, eraser, stamp, and apple, orange, cherry. This is clearly a difficult task, and without norms it is difficult to interpret the patient's poor performance. Nevertheless, the patient performed well on this task when the choices were given orally, suggesting that the conceptual difficulty

per se cannot account for his poor performance sorting the visual stimuli. Gil et al. report a similar finding with their subject: She did poorly at
sorting pictures based on "metaphorical" association unless they were
named aloud for her.

The neuropathology of optic aphasia shows a fair degree of uniform-
ity. All cases appear to have unilateral left posterior lesions; in cases with
sufficient localizing evidence the damage seems to include the occipital
cortex and white matter.

4.6 Relation Between Associative Agnosia and Optic Aphasia

Associative agnosics and optic aphasics share certain characteristics,
and these similarities have led some authors to classify them as a single
syndrome (Geschwind, 1965), or to suggest that they differ only in degree
rather than in kind (e.g., Bauer and Rubens, 1985; Kertesz, 1987). Indeed,
the most prominent characteristic of each is shared by the other: They
cannot name visually presented stimuli, even though their naming of
tactile and auditory stimuli is relatively unimpaired. In addition, both
types of patients demonstrate apparently good elementary visual perception, as measured by their ability to copy drawings that they cannot
name and describe the visual appearance of objects. However, there are
also several important differences between these two types of patients:
Optic aphasics can indicate their recognition of a visual stimulus by
sorting it with other stimuli of the same category, whereas associative
agnosics cannot. Some optic aphasics can gesture an appropriate pantomime to a visual stimulus, whereas associative agnosics cannot. In their
everyday life, optic aphasics are not described as impaired, whereas associative agnosics are often noted to be handicapped by an inability to
recognize people, common objects, and locales. Associative agnosics
show tremendous sensitivity to the visual quality of the stimulus, identifying real objects more accurately than photographs and photographs
more accurately than drawings, and identifying visual stimuli better at
long exposure durations than at short ones, whereas optic aphasics are
insensitive to this task dimension. The nature of the errors made by these
two kinds of patients differs as well: Visual errors predominate in
associative agnosia, whereas semantic errors and perseverations predominate in optic aphasia. Note that these differences are not differences
in degree, such that optic aphasics have the same characteristics as
agnosics but in milder form. Optic aphasics show *more* perseveration and
semantic errors than associative agnosics. At roughly equivalent levels of
naming peformance, associative agnosics are affected by visual stimulus
quality, whereas optic aphasics are not. In summary, there are several

characteristics that occur with great consistency within just one or the other of these groups of patients, justifying their separation into distinct categories.

Earlier it was mentioned that there has been some confusion in the literature between these two categories of patients. In some instances this has come about because of an author's principled decision to collapse the categories of associative agnosia and optic aphasia, as when Bauer and Rubens (1985) refer to the case of Lhermitte and Beauvois as a case of associative agnosia. In other instances it appears to reflect a lack of awareness of the differences between these categories. Let us use the framework of distinguishing characteristics just developed to evaluate two such recent cases.

Ferro and Santos (1984) published a detailed report entitled "Associative Visual Agnosia: A Case study." Included in their description of the patient was the observation that "When faced with an object he could not recognize visually and asked to pantomime its use, he almost always succeeded" (p. 125), like some of the optic aphasics described earlier, and unlike any other associative agnosics. Furthermore, his sorting of visually presented objects was reasonably good (p. 129: 80 percent correct for objects) and not very different from his performance on the analogous test with spoken words rather than visual stimuli (p. 127: 90 percent correct). Recall that several of the optic aphasics performed less than perfectly on this type of task. Like the optic aphasics just described, and in contrast to the associative agnosics, his naming errors were most often perseverations, and more often anomic or semantic than visual (p. 126). In addition, like the optic aphasics, but unlike the associative agnosics, his ability to name pictures was relatively insensitive to perceptual factors such as size and inspection time (p. 126). It is of course possible that some degree of associative agnosia was superimposed on the optic aphasia in this case, but the latter syndrome appears to predominate.

Similarly, the patient of Caplan and Hedley-Whyte (1974), presented as a case of pure alexia with associative visual agnosia in an article entitled "Cuing and Memory Dysfunction in Alexia without Agraphia: A Case Report," appears to have more in common with cases of optic aphasia than alexia or associative object agnosia. In naming visual stimuli, she produces the same "conduites d'approache" or homing-in behavior described by Lhermitte and Beauvois and Gil et al. (1985), arriving at the correct name after several near misses. For example, when shown a picture of a bus, she said, "A map, no, I know it, of course, ought to be able to say it. Not a map . . . It's a road, you use it on a road . . . [Examiner: Is it a bus?] It could be a bus, yes, yes, that's what it is, a bus." A picture of a bathtub elicited "It's for water, you measure with it ["measure" is a perseveration from a previous response], a sink, no, you have it near a sink, like a faucet, a drain, it has another name, I know. [Examiner: What do you do with it?] Take a bath in it." This patient also showed florid perseveration. More central to the distinction between optic aphasia and associative agnosia is evidence concerning recognition of visual stimuli that cannot be named. Although the authors did not test recognition of objects or pictures nonverbally, they did observe evidence that the patient was able to recognize letters and words that she could not name. For example, when shown disoriented letters of the alphabet, she quickly put them in the correct orientation. Although low-level visual cues, such as symmetry and axes of elongation, might be of some help in this task, one could not use them to distinguish between upright and inverted letters. The dissociation between her naming ability and her recognition ability was also evident when she correctly ordered printed letters of the alphabet, despite misnaming the letters aloud as she proceeded. Finally, she was able to complete the letters in a word (e.g., if the "A" in "CAT" were missing its crossbar) and eliminate superfluous letters in a word (e.g., cover up the "XE" in "XEDOG"), again without being able to name the words.

The idea that associative agnosia and optic aphasia are distinct syndromes with different characteristics does not rule out the possibility that patients could suffer a combination of them. As already mentioned, the case of Ferro and Santos (1984) may have had some associative agnosia overlaying his optic aphasia, although characteristics of the latter seemed to predominate. The famous case of Lissauer (1890), which prompted him to draw the apperceptive/associative distinction, appears to have had a mixture of problems. Lissauer declined to categorize his case as apperceptive or associative, as elements of both were present. The frequent semantic errors and perseverations made by this patient suggest that optic aphasia was also present.

Chapter 5

Interpreting the Associative Agnosias in terms of
Theories of Normal Object Recognition

5.1 Associative Object Agnosia

5.1.1 Minimalist models of object recognition: Disconnection accounts of agnosia

An influential attempt at interpreting associative agnosia in terms of a comprehensive theoretical framework was made by Geschwind in part II of his 1965 article, "Disconnexion Syndromes in Animal and Man." In this article, Geschwind elaborates on the ideas of Dejerine (e.g., 1892), Liepmann (e.g., 1900), and other nineteenth century neurologists concerning the role of neuroanatomical disconnections in explaining a wide range of neuropsychological deficits. According to these writers, many apparently high-level and selective neuropsychological deficits can be explained without having to postulate damage to "centers" that normally carry out these lost high-level functions. Instead, they can be explained by patterns of disconnection among a relatively smaller set of intact centers with relatively simpler functions. The appeal of such explanations lies in their parsimony and in their ability to relate psychological function directly to neuroanatomy.

Geschwind (1965) proposed that visual agnosia was not caused by the loss of some "visual recognition ability," but rather by the disconnection of intact visual areas from language areas. According to Geschwind, most cases of associative agnosia are simply cases of visual-verbal disconnection. Patients' introspections that they cannot recognize objects, or that objects look strange to them, which would seem to indicate an impairment in visual recognition per se, are explained as confabulations made in response to the unusual condition of visual-verbal disconnection, much as aphasic or dysarthric patients may attribute their speech difficulties to a dry mouth or poorly fitting dentures. The misnaming of objects as visually similar objects, which would seem to indicate dysfunction within the visual processing domain, is explained in terms of partial residual connection.

Although disconnection accounts of neuropsychological phenomena are sometimes said to be accounts of neuropathology, and not psychology (e.g., Friedman and Alexander, 1984; Patterson and Kay, 1982), Geschwind's interpretation of agnosia is clearly an hypothesis about the functional architecture of visual object recognition as well as its neuroanatomic instantiation. That Geschwind was not limiting his theorizing to the neuropathogenesis of agnosia, but was concerned with psychological processes, is apparent when he states that "I believe in fact that there is no single faculty of 'recognition' but that the term covers the totality of all the associations aroused by an object. Phrased another way, we 'manifest recognition' by responding appropriately; to the extent that any appropriate response occurs, we have shown 'recognition'. But this view abolishes the notion of a unitary step of 'recognition'; instead, there are multiple parallel processes of appropriate response to a stimulus" (p. 587). This view of recognition fit in well with the behaviorist agenda of replacing mentalistic terms with sets of stimulus-response pairings, which was dominant in the psychology of the time (e.g., see Skinner, 1965).

By dispensing with a "faculty" of recognition, Geschwind can account quite parsimoniously for some of the major characteristics of agnosia. However, a slightly finer-grained view of agnosia reveals several phenomena that are problematic for Geschwind's disconnection account. These are essentially the differences between optic aphasia and associative agnosia discussed in the last chapter. If associative agnosia were nothing more than a visual-verbal disconnection, then agnosics should be able to express their recognition of objects nonverbally, for example, by gesturing or by sorting together objects that are semantically related. However, associative agnosics cannot do these things. Another difference between the predictions of a visual-verbal disconnection and the behavior of associative agnosics concerns the ability of these patients to interact normally with objects seen in everyday life. Although Geschwind asserts that agnosics do interact normally with the visual world, as one would expect if their deficit were one of visual naming rather than visual recognition, he does not cite specific findings to support this assertion. The observations described in the last chapter show that agnosic patients are frequently impaired in such nonverbal interactions with the visual world as finding their way about, eating, dressing, and socializing. Although an agnosic patient would be expected to benefit to some degree from the availability of context in familiar surroundings, and to make inferences about the identity of objects based on such context, this is not inconsistent with a deficit in recognition per se. In fact, Riddoch and Humphreys (1987a) investigated the effect of context on an agnosic patient's ability to identify drawings of objects and found that context allowed the patient to improve his performance, but that the improvement appeared to be achieved by means of postrecognition inferences. A final difficulty for the visual-verbal disconnection account of agnosia stems from dissociations among different types of agnosia. If visual input is cut off from language centers, then why should different patients be more or less impaired at the naming of faces, objects, colors, or printed words? Such dissociations make sense if category-specific visual representations are destroyed. To explain them in terms of inter-ruptions in category-specific pathways between the visual and verbal areas is not altogether implausible, but it does seem to imply that category-specific representations already exist within the visual areas, in which case much of the theoretical parsimony of the disconnection account has been lost.

A different kind of attempt to account for associative agnosia within the disconnection framework has been suggested by Albert, Soffer, Silverberg and Reches (1979); Bauer, (1982), and Gomori and Hawryluk (1984). These authors propose that associative visual agnosia is caused by bilateral disconnection of the visual areas from the medial temporal structures important for memory, such as the hippocampus and amygdala. The idea behind this proposal seems to be that visual recognition ability involves both vision and memory, and a disconnection between visual and memory centers would therefore disrupt visual recognition ability. This account is consistent with the neuropathology in many cases of associative agnosia, as the bilateral occipitotemporal lesions generally encompass both gray and white matter (the latter connecting visual and medial temporal areas). However, there is at least one case that has come to autopsy in which the damage was confined to occipito-temporal gray matter (Cambier et al., 1980), suggesting that a loss of "processing centers" and/or representations, rather than connections, is at fault.

A more fundamental problem with this account is that the medial temporal structures in question are primarily involved in the acquisition of new memories, not the storage of old memories (e.g., see Squire, 1987). Therefore, a disconnection between visual areas and medial temporal areas would be expected to produce a visual modality-specific deficit in new learning, and not an inability to recognize long-familiar visual stimuli. Such a visual learning deficit has been described in two cases of bilateral occipitotemporal damage by Ross (1980). Both patients per-formed poorly on tests of visual recognition memory after only a few minutes had elapsed since stimulus presentation. In contrast, they per-formed well on tests of tactile, auditory-verbal, and auditory-nonverbal memory, consistent with the hypothesized specificity of the neu-roanatomic disconnection. Although one of the patients was prosopag-nosic, the other was reportedly not agnosic. Further evidence that a visual-medial temporal disconnection could not be the cause of associative agnosia comes from the study of amnesia after medial temporal damage. Such patients are not agnosic, despite the fact that they are no more able to send information from the visual to the medial temporal memory areas than a patient with a lesion disconnecting these areas would be.

The shortcomings of the disconnection accounts of agnosia have led to other conceptualizations of visual recognition in neuropsychology, in which a specific "recognition" stage is posited. Although these explanations have less parsimony than the disconnection explanations, in which "recognition" is merely the interaction between visual perceptual (as opposed to visual memory) processes on the one hand and amodal (as opposed to visual) memory and language processes on the other, they are better able to account for the full range of phenomena in associative agnosia. There are two different accounts of associative visual agnosia that include an identifiable "recognition" stage in visual object recognition, distinct from visual perception *per se* and memory and language *per se*.

5.1.2 Symbolic search models of object recognition: Agnosia as a loss of stored visual representations

According to this view of the recognition process, visual perception proceeds through some relatively abstract representation of the stimulus, which is then compared against stored memory representations of stimuli in the same abstract format until a match is found. Humphreys and Riddoch (1987a) offer an analogy with finding a book in a library: The stimulus representation is like the title written on a slip of paper that one carries to the book stacks. This is compared with the titles written on the spines of the books. These latter titles are analogous to the stored long-term visual memory representations. When a match is found, recognition has occurred, and all of the knowledge associated with the stored representation (the information in the books, in this analogy) can be accessed. Figure 23 shows a model that embodies this view of visual object recognition, taken from the work of Humphreys and Riddoch.

This view of visual object recognition is quite compatible with traditional computational architectures for memory, including the "architectures" of libraries and paper filing systems as well as symbol-manipulating computers. Perhaps for this reason, it has appealed to many neuropsychologists seeking an account of associative agnosia. Efron (1968) points out that many early authors explained agnosia by a "loss of the 'stored visual memories' or 'engrams' of objects," citing Dejerine (1914), von Monakow (1914), and Nielsen (1936). The same idea has been put in

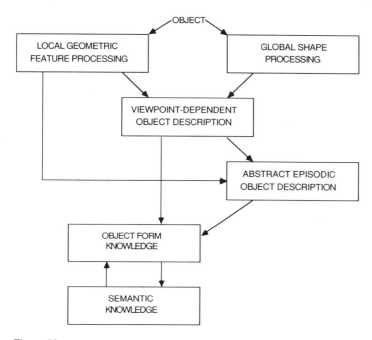

Figure 23
Information-processing framework suggested by Humphreys and Riddoch (1987b) for understanding visual object recognition and its disorders.

slightly different terms by many other writers. For example, Brown (1972), speaks of the associative agnosic deficit as affecting "the matching of signal to trace" (p. 219). Damasio (1985) attributes at least some cases of prosopagnosia to a destruction of stored "templates" (p. 263). Mesulam (1985) also cites the contribution of the "destruction of previously formed templates" in explaining object agnosia (p. 18).

Let us examine just what would constitute evidence for or against this account of agnosia, and the functional architecture of visual object recognition that it entails. If there are cases of agnosia due to a loss of stored long-term visual memory representations, then they should display normal visual perception at all levels of representation, because the derived stimulus representations are distinct from the representations hypothesized to have been destroyed. We thus return to the issue of whether perception is ever normal in associative agnosia and, more importantly, whether the abnormalities that have been noted are causal of the agnosia. Five general kinds of evidence on the status of visual perception in associative agnosia were reviewed in the last chapter: The slavish manner with which patients copy drawings and perform matching tasks; the visual nature of their identification errors; the sensitivity of their recognition performance to the visual quality of stimuli; patients' introspections that their vision is abnormal, and the results of various experimental tasks designed to test visual perception (feature integration, closure tasks, and discriminating possible from impossible figures). How do each of these types of evidence bear on the hypothesis that agnosia is caused by a loss of stored visual memory representations?

A preliminary comment that applies to all of the relevant evidence concerns the problem of making inferences in neuropsychology from associations between deficits. A case of associative agnosia in which perception was tested in all of the ways mentioned above and found to be intact would constitute a dissociation between recognition ability and perceptual ability, and would thereby confirm the hypothesis that damage to the stored visual memories was the cause of the agnosia. Unfortunately, the absence of such a case, in other words an association between recognition deficits and perceptual deficits, is ambiguous. It is certainly consistent with the hypothesis that associative agnosia is caused by perceptual impairments rather than impairment in stored visual memory representations. The problem is that it is also consistent with the hypothesis that associative agnosia is caused by impairment in stored visual memory representations, and that for theoretically uninteresting reasons (e.g., neuroanatomical propinquity of perceptual processing centers and stored visual memories) perception happens to be impaired whenever the visual memory stores are impaired. This problem is compounded by the fact that only a relatively small number of cases of associative agnosia have been reported, and even fewer have been properly examined for perceptual abnormalities.

In addition to these very general considerations about inferences from neuropsychological associations, there are additional considerations particular to each type of evidence. Visual errors, that is, the misidentification of an object as a similar-looking object, might seem to imply that perception is impaired. Furthermore, they might seem particularly relevant to the issue of whether the perceptual abnormalities cause the agnosia, as opposed to being merely superimposed upon it, because they are manifest during failed attempts at object recognition, and not just on visual tests unrelated to object recognition. Unfortunately, visual errors can be accounted for equally well by the alternative hypothesis, that visual perception is normal and visual memory stores are impaired. If stored visual memories were damaged (e.g., a certain number of visual features lost, in the context of a feature-based theory), they would presumably become less discriminable from one another, and an incoming stimulus representation would therefore be more likely to "match" with the stored representation of a similar-looking object. Similarly, the finding that recognition abilities of agnosic patients are drastically affected by perceptual degradation of the stimulus does not necessarily implicate a perceptual locus for the agnosic impairment: It is conceivable that degradation of the stimulus would make it harder to obtain the proper match with stored representations if those stored representations were themselves degraded.

Evidence from copying tasks and matching tasks is somewhat more decisive. The fact that associative agnosics copy and compare drawings slowly and slavishly is consistent with the hypothesis that they see them abnormally. Furthermore, these tasks do not, on the face of things, require the use of hypothesized stored visual memories. Of course, it is likely that some degree of top-down support for copying and matching normally comes from knowledge of the stimuli. Nevertheless, the impairment does not seem to be completely attributable to the absence of top-down support. Even when copying or matching meaningless visual stimuli, for which they have no stored visual memories, normal subjects do not adopt the slavish, line by line copying strategy that is characteristic of associative visual agnosics.

In the few cases described earlier in which experimental tasks have been devised to assess the perceptual abilities of associative agnosic patients, the results have added further support to the existence of serious perceptual impairments in these cases (Humphreys and Riddoch, 1987; Levine and Calvanio, 1989; Mendez, 1988; Ratcliff and Newcombe, 1982). The tasks used in two of these have little, if any, reliance on stored visual memories: searching for simple target shapes in a feature integration task, and discriminating possible from impossible abstract shapes. Although in Levine and Calvanio's study the stimuli were meaningful words and objects, there are additional reasons to believe that visual memory was not the source of the patient's problems in these tasks. First, when unable to recognize the object or word in a closure task, he was also unable to indicate its contour, implying that he was unable to perceive the stimulus. Second, his agnosia did not extend to written material, implying that his visual memory for written material was intact, but he nevertheless performed poorly on closure tasks in which the stimuli were words. It is also worth mentioning that patients' introspections are consistent with the hypothesis that their visual perception is impaired, adding some additional support to the more objective forms of evidence just reviewed.

Within the limitations inherent in making inferences from an association observed in a relatively small number of cases, the available data suggest that perception is not normal in associative agnosia. There appears to be a rather consistent pattern of impairment manifest in the way in which these patients copy and compare drawings, and their performance on other tasks as well as their introspections also indicate that perception is not normal. It therefore seems unlikely that associative agnosia is caused by damage to stored visual memory representations.

The implications of this conclusion for the functional architecture of visual object recognition concern the existence of two types of high-level visual representation, the stored visual memories and the derived visual stimulus representations. If there were cases of associative agnosia with intact perception, this would be interpretable as a loss of stored visual memories with intact derived stimulus representations, and this in turn would imply the existence of these two separate types of high-level visual representation. Given the absence of such a case, we are led to consider a different view of visual object recognition, based on a very different computational architecture.

5.1.3 Massively parallel constraint-satisfaction models of object recognition: Agnosia as loss of knowledge how to perceive objects

In the computational architecture for memory search described in the previous section, a representation of the stimulus is derived and then compared to stored representations that are identifiable and distinct from the stimulus representation. As in the library analogy, in which there is one copy of the call number on a slip of paper and one copy on the spine of the book, so in this architecture more generally there are two distinct representational tokens of the object being recognized: the one derived from the stimulus and the one that is stored. Recent work in computational vision has focussed on a very different architecture for visual recognition, called variously "cooperative computation," "massively parallel computation," "parallel distributed processing," "connectionism," or computation by "constraint satisfaction." In these systems, one need not postulate separate representational tokens for the stimulus and the stored memory. Because these systems seem to provide a promising framework for explaining the relations between perception and memory in agnosia, some general background about them will be reviewed here.

In massively parallel contraint-satisfaction systems, the stimulus representation consists of a pattern of activation across a set of highly interconnected neuronlike units. The extent to which activation in one unit causes activation in the other units to which it is connected depends upon the connection strengths, or weights, between the units. As in the McClelland and Rumelhart word perception model discussed in section 3.3.1, units representing consisent hypotheses tend to activate each other, whereas units representing inconsistent hypotheses tend to inhibit each other (that is, increased activation in one leads to a decrease in the activation of the other). This is accomplished by having positive "weights" on the connections between units representing consistent hypotheses and negative weights on the connections between units representing inconsistent hypotheses. Memory representations consist of the pattern of weights, or connection strengths, among all of the units.

Presenting a stimulus to the system results in an initial pattern of activation levels across the units, such that some units will be highly activated, some less so, and some not at all. At this point the activation levels of each unit will begin to change under the influence of the other units to which they are connected and according to the weights on those connections. In effect, each unit is satisfying as best it can the constraints on its activation level imposed by its neighbors' activation levels and the strengths of its connections to the neighboring units. Eventually, as a result of these local interactions, the network as a whole "settles" into a stable state that represents the most consistent set of hypotheses about the input. In terms of the problem of visual object recognition, the network will seek a state that is maximally consistent with the activation from the stimulus and the knowledge of object appearances encoded in the connection strengths. It thus arrives at an interpretation of the stimulus that combines information from the stimulus and from previous perceptual experience.

One of the strengths of this computational architecture is that it can find solutions to problems in which many different types of constraints apply simultaneously (McClelland, Rumelhart, and Hinton, 1986). This characterizes the central problem in object recognition, in which the retinal image of the object is determined jointly by the true shape of the object and various confounding factors such as viewing angle, lighting, occlusion, and so on, and the goal is to recover the true shape of the object from the image. This involves finding an interpretation of the image that satisfies the constraints of being consistent with a possible true object shape viewed under some mutually consistent set of viewing conditions (perspective, lighting, occlusion). To take the relatively simple example of block letter recognition, a vertical line segment could be the upright bar of an "I" viewed at an orientation, or the cross-bar of an "H" viewed at a 90° orientation, or many other possible combinations of letter-features and letter-orientations. When such a feature is visible in a stimulus, our choice of interpretation for that feature, and hence our identification of the stimulus, depends upon the other features visible at the same time. In particular, the interpretation of all of the different features must satisfy the constraint of being consistent with a single letter at a single orientation (known as the "viewpoint consistency constraint," Lowe, 1987). Hinton (1981) has developed a model that accomplishes this by simultaneously taking into account the constraints that relate all possible views of all possible objects and settling into a representation of the viewpoint and object that best explains the retinal visual input. A representative portion of the model is shown in figure 24. A brief description of the workings of the model follows, with the hope of giving interested readers a "feel" for computation by constraint satisfaction in the domain of object recognition.

The stimulus activates a pattern of input units, called the "retina-based units" (which represent the features of the letter in retina-based coordinates, i.e., relative to the viewer's gaze). The retina-based units activate all object-based features with which they are consistent. For example, the retina-based unit for a vertical line segment will activate the object-based unit for a vertical line segment (because it is consistent with such an object

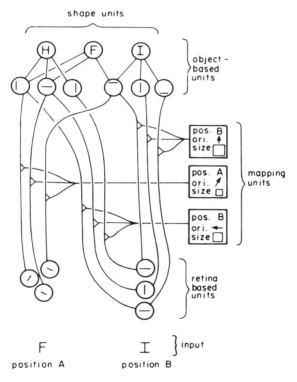

Figure 24
Part of Hinton's (1981) model of object recognition. See text for an explanation.

feature if the object were upright) and the object-based unit for a horizontal line segment (because it is consistent with such an object-based feature if the object were being viewed at a 90° orientation). But, it will not activate any curved object-based feature units, for example, because it is not consistent with them. Object-based feature units then activate the object units with which they are consistent. In addition, activation flows top-down, with object units activating the object-based feature units with which they are consistent, and object-based feature units activating the retina-based feature units with which they are consistent, and inhibition flows between inconsistent object units. Of course, the relations between retina-based features and object-based features are only weakly constrained; although a straight line segment retina-based feature cannot be consistent with a curved line segment object-based feature, it is consistent with a large number of different straight line segment object-based features. Stronger, and therefore more useful, constraints involve a three-way relation between retina-based units, object-based units, and "mapping units," which represent the different possible orientations of the object. If any two of the three properties, retina-based feature, object-based feature, and object orientation, are known, the third can be deduced because the other two constrain it fully. The triangle-shaped connections in figure 24 represent the fact that joint activity in the retina and object-based units activates the "mapping units" representing the object orientations that relate the two. Returning to the earlier example, activation of the retina-based unit for a vertical line segment and the object-based unit for a vertical line segment will cause the vertical mapping unit to become active, representing the hypothesis that the letter is vertically oriented with respect to the viewer, whereas activation of the retina-based unit for a vertical line segment and the object-based unit for a horizontal line segment will cause the 90° mapping unit to become active, representing the hypothesis that the letter is at a 90° orientation with respect to the viewer. The constraints embodied in the connection-strengths among the units, along with the input activation, are generally sufficient to ensure that the system will eventually settle into a stable state in which a single object unit and mapping unit are active. This corresponds to having identified the object and its orientation.

In massively parallel models of object recognition, the distinction between the derived stimulus representation and the stored representation dissolves: Depending upon the connection strengths, incoming activation will settle into one stable pattern or another, corresponding to the perceived identity of the object. There is no process whereby the incoming pattern of activation is "matched against" another pattern of activation. One could say of this type of system that it *sees* things differently depending upon the memories it has embodied in its connection strengths. The available evidence on the relation between object perception and object recognition in agnosia is compatible with the effects of damage to massively parallel object recognition systems, in that memory cannot be altered without altering perception. According to this view, what has been impaired in agnosia is either the pattern of weights among the units, or the units themselves, such that the network settles into incomplete or incorrect interpretations of the stimulus.

5.2 Prosopagnosia

5.2.1 Stored facial templates versus constraint satisfaction

The issue just discussed, of whether stored visual memories can be damaged without affecting the perceptual analysis of visual stimuli, is relevant to the interpretation of prosopagnosia as well as general associative object agnosia. In this case, the question is, Do we have a stored "library" of visual face representations, against which incoming face representations are compared, such that just the "library" representations can be damaged? Such a view is common in the cognitive psychology and neuropsychology literatures on face recognition. For example, the influential model of Bruce and Young (1986, pp. 311–312), shown in figure 25, contains a module labelled "structural encoding," which constructs an abstract structural code for the incoming stimulus face, and a separate module labelled "face recognition units," which contains stored structural codes of known faces. Damasio (1985) invokes a similar framework when he speaks of prosopagnosia as destruction of the stored "facial template system". The kinds of evidence relevant to this issue are essentially those reviewed in the previous section: Evidence about the quality of perception in these patients. The most direct test of the relevant perceptual abilities in these patients comes from the Benton and Van Allen test of facial discrimination, and, as already discussed, there is no documented case of prosopagnosia in which the patient performs this test normally, in terms of both speed and accuracy. Therefore, available evidence is more supportive of a constraint satisfaction architecture for face recognition than of a "stored template" system.

5.2.2 Category-specific recognition systems? Qualitative and quantitative differences between prosopagnosia and object agnosia

Whether prosopagnosia and across-the-board object agnosia differ in degree or kind is an issue of debate in neuropsychology, which has implications for the functional architecture of normal vision. There are

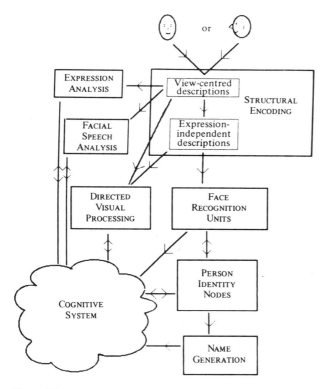

Figure 25
Information-processing framework suggested by Bruce and Young (1986) for understanding face recognition and its disorders.

three general accounts of the relation between the two syndromes. One of these could be called a "differential difficulty" account. According to this type of account, there is but a single system for visual recognition. If the damage to this single system is slight, then the patient will be agnosic only for stimuli that are normally most "difficult" to recognize. It is argued, not implausibly, that faces, animals, plants, buildings, and so on are "difficult". Several writers have endorsed this type of account (Brown, 1972; Gloning, Gloning, Jellinger, and Quatember, 1970; Humphreys and Riddoch, 1987a; Mesulam, 1985). For example, Gloning et al. suggest that "prosopagnosia is an attenuated form of visual object agnosia, and differs from it in degree rather than in kind" (p. 203).

In favor of the "differential difficulty" account, it takes an extremely parsimonious view of the functional architecture of visual object recognition. Prosopagnosia and object agnosia can both be explained by postulating different severities of damage to a single system. Against this type of account, there is no independent evidence that the stimuli that prosopagnosics cannot recognize are truly harder for normal subjects to recognize than the stimuli that prosopagnosics can recognize. We are asked to accept this based on its intuitive plausibility. In order to test the "differential difficulty" hypothesis directly, one would need to measure the performance of prosopagnosics *relative to normal subjects* at recognizing the affected and unaffected categories of stimuli. If prosopagnosics were found to be equally impaired, with respect to normal subjects, at recognizing both faces, animals, etc., on the one hand and common objects on the other, then this would confirm the differential difficulty account. In contrast, if prosopagnosics were selectively impaired at recognizing faces, animals, etc., relative to normal subjects, this would disconfirm the differential difficulty account. Unfortunately, such an experiment would be interpretable only if normal subjects were not performing at ceiling in the object recognition task, and perhaps because of this methodological obstacle, no such test has been reported. There are two recent experiments that have some indirect relevance to this issue, however. One experiment involves visual imagery, rather than recognition, but is presumably relevant to the issue of the functional architecture of visual object recognition given evidence of shared representations for visual imagery and higher visual perception (Farah, 1988). In addition, normal subjects are not invariably at ceiling on imagery tasks, making it possible to scale the performance of a brain-damaged subject against that of normal subjects. In this experiment, we (Farah, Hammond, Mehta, and Ratcliff, 1989) measured the performance of the agnosic patient L.H. and normal subjects on a test of visual imagery for living things (i.e., categories of stimuli among those that prosopagnosics find difficult: animals and plants) and nonliving things (i.e., categories of stimuli that prosopagnosics can generally recognize: tools, furniture, musical instruments, etc.). L.H., whose agnosia is not limited to faces and living things but who is particularly impaired at recognizing these categories of stimuli, was also impaired, relative to normal subjects, at imaging the living things. More to the point, his performance was significantly more impaired on living than on nonliving things, relative to normal subjects'. This implies that the patient's selective impairment in imagery for living things cannot be accounted for by the "differential difficulty" of imaging living things compared to nonliving things.

A second study addressed the ability of two such patients to recognize line drawings of living and nonliving things (Farah, McMullen and Meyer, submitted). L.H. and M.B. were shown the 260 drawings from the Snodgrass and Vanderwart corpus on several occasions, and the proportion of each subjects' correct identification responses for each drawing was submitted to a logit regression analysis. As independent factors in the analysis, we included normal subjects' ratings of the visual complexity, familiarity and typicality of the depiction of each picture, as well as its degree of similarity to the most similar other object they can imagine. We also included categorical variables denoting whether the standard name for the picture was a "basic object level" term (e.g., "chair") or a more specific term (e.g., "rocking chair;" for discussion of the possible relevance of this factor, see below), and whether the depicted item was living or nonliving. The factors influencing each subject's recognition performance were almost the same, and in each case the living-nonliving distinction remained highly predictive of recognition performance even with the other variables in the analysis.

Further evidence against the "differential difficulty" explanation comes from the double dissociation between face recognition and object recognition: There are agnosic patients who are impaired at recognizing objects but show little or no impairment for faces (e.g., Feinberg, Gonzalez-Rothi, and Heilman, 1986; Hecaen and Ajuriaguerra, 1956; McCarthy and Warrington, 1986; Pillon, Signoret and Lhermitte, 1981; see table 1 for others). If there is a single visual recognition faculty, and we explain the apparent selectivity of prosopagnosia by saying that faces, animals, etc., are harder to recognize than most common objects, then how do we explain agnosia for objects with spared face recognition?

A second possibility was proposed by Faust (1955) and championed more recently by Damasio, Damasio, and Van Hoesen (1982). This account distinguishes between the process of recognizing the general category to which an object belongs, and the process of recognizing the specific exemplar within the category, and could thus be called a "within versus between category" account. Prosopagnosics are said to have an impairment in distinguishing among objects within a category, but not among objects between categories. That is, they can recognize that a face is a face, a bird is a bird, a building is a building, and so on. What they cannot recognize is *which* face, animal, building, etc., they are viewing. In the words of Damasio, et al., "Recognition of the generic class to which the stimulus belongs presents no difficulty, but recognition of an individual member of that class, whose identity had previously been learned, is impaired. But it has not been noted that if instead of being asked to identify, say, a 'book' or a 'chair', the patient is asked 'whose book' or 'whose chair' it is, the patient will fail to answer . . . We contend that the emphasis on the dissociation between facial recognition and object recognition is misleading. The two performances, as traditionally elicited by examiners, are different . . . The valid dissociation is between the recognition of the generic conceptual class to which the object belongs and the recognition of the historical context of a given object [i.e., the individual identity of the object] vis a vis the subject" (p. 337). Note that this account is distinct from the "differential difficulty" account described earlier. There is no necessary relation between the level of the category hierarchy at which visual recognition takes place and the difficulty (for normal subjects) of recognition. Damasio (1985) points this out by saying that "Patients with prosopagnosia can perceive and recognize accurately many stimuli that are visually more complex than human faces" (p 133).

The "within versus between category" account has considerable appeal, as it seems to explain many of the phenomena of prosopagnosia in terms of a simple distinction between hierarchical levels of memory representation. Although it is less parsimonious in its implicit model of visual object recognition than the "differential difficulty" account, as it distinguishes between visual recognition processes needed to arrive at a category-level identification and others needed to arrive at a within-category identification, it nevertheless manages to avoid the seemingly less palatable interpretation of prosopagnosia, in terms of recognition systems that are specialized for particular kinds of stimuli (e.g., faces, animals, buildings, etc.). Just the same, problems remain for this type of account. One problem is conceptual: How is the "category" level specified? There are many categories into which a particular object can be classed, covering a wide range of specificity to generality. For any given stimulus that prosopagnosics can or cannot identify, we can always find some category for which it will be true that the patient can make between-category discriminations and not within-category discriminations. One need only find the most specific level of category that the prosopagnosic can reliably use for the object, and then go down one level in the hierarchy to find the selective "within-category deficit." Another way of demonstrating the surplus degrees of freedom in this account is to point out that we can find categories for which prosopagnosics will show good within-category discrimination (e.g., furniture) or bad between-category discrimination (e.g., Yellow-naped Amazon Parrot versus Panama Parrot). Damasio and colleagues are apparently relying on certain intuitions about the relevant category level, perhaps akin to the concept of "basic object level category" in cognitive psychology (Rosch, Mervis, Gray, Johnson, and Boyes-Braem, 1976). However, without some explicit constraints on the category level, this account is not explanatory.

Even using our intuitions about the appropriate category level, problems remain with the "within- versus between-category" account. In general, prosopagnosic patients do not seem to have trouble making within-category discriminations for many seemingly "basic object" categories. Although Damasio et al. (1982) attribute this to lack of appropriate testing, it must be admitted that prosopagnosics spontaneously complain of their difficulty recognizing faces, animals, cars, and so on, but do not complain of difficulty recognizing their own books, chairs, or other subordinate exemplars of "basic object level" categories. Furthermore, to the limited degree that this hypothesis has been directly tested, the data have failed to support it. Recall that De Renzi's (1986) case 4 was able to select his own razor, necktie, and other articles from sets of similar-looking ones, and that the two cases studied by Farah, McMullen and Meyer showed greater impairment with living things even when category level was accounted for.

A third possibility is that the visual recognition system does indeed treat certain stimuli, the ones that are difficult for prosopagnosics, differently from other stimuli. That is, there is a separate subsystem that is important for recognizing faces, and perhaps, to a lesser extent, for recognizing animals, foods, buildings, makes of automobile, and so on. This type of account could be called a "stimulus-specific recognition systems" account. It is clearly less parsimonious than the "differential difficulty" account. It also seems less parsimonious than the "within- versus between-category" account, in that we have independent reasons for believing that certain levels of categorization are cognitively and perceptually primary or privileged (Rosch, et al., 1976). Another drawback of the "stimulus-specific recognition systems" account is that, although it certainly fits the available data well, it is equally capable of fitting any arbitrary data: Whatever prosopagnosics cannot recognize can be assumed to be in the set of stimuli normally processed by the hypothesized special subsystem. In other words, this account appears to have the drawback of being ad hoc as well as unparsimonious. Let us consider how serious these drawbacks are.

One mitigating consideration is that there is independent evidence of brain mechanisms specialized for recognizing the types of stimuli that prosopagnosics find difficult. Perhaps the most remarkable findings along these lines come from single unit recordings in monkeys, which have revealed a population of neurons in the temporal lobe that respond selectively to faces. For example, Perrett, Rolls, and Caan (1982) found that just under 10 percent of the 500 cells they sampled in the superior temporal sulcus (STS) of the macaque monkey responded to faces, and not to other stimuli. Desimone, Albright, Gross and Bruce (1984) found that 34 percent of the 50 cells that they sampled in the same area showed selective responses to faces. Baylis, Rolls, and Leonard (1985) identified 44 face-selective cells in the superior temporal sulcus and studied their responses to different faces. They found that 77 percent of these cells reliably responded more to certain faces than to others. This last finding is perhaps most relevant to the issue of prosopagnosia, as it concerns the ability of the cells to discriminate between faces.

In addition to their selective responses to faces, the STS cells have other properties that suggest a role in face recognition. Like normal human observers, these cells are able to "recognize" pictures of faces under conditions of changed illumination, spatial frequency filtering, change of expression, and deletion of a feature (Desimone, et al., 1984; Rolls, 1984; Rolls and Baylis, 1986). Also like normal human observers, the cells do not recognize the identity of a face whose features have been rearranged (e.g., nose above eyes, mouth on side) (Desimone, et al., 1984; Perrett et al., 1982). One apparent divergence between the response properties of these cells and of the visual recognition system of intact humans is the absence of an "inversion" effect. Whereas normal humans cannot reliably recognize inverted faces (Yin, 1969), the face-sensitive cells in macaque monkeys respond as vigorously to inverted faces as they do to upright faces (Desimone et al., 1984). The findings of Bruce (1982) help to explain this inconsistency: He found that macaques recognize inverted faces as well as they recognize upright faces. This is probably the result of the greater range of viewing angles experienced by monkeys looking at faces than by humans. Consistent with this interpretation are recent recordings from sheep temporal cortex showing face-selective cells that respond only to upright faces (Kendrick and Baldwin, 1987).

In trying to relate the single unit recording literature to prosopagnosia, one wants to know about single unit responses to stimuli other than faces that prosopagnosics are unable to recognize. Unfortunately, there has been relatively little systematic investigation of the responses of these cells to objects other than faces, and none that specifically concerns the subset of nonface objects with which prosopagnosics have difficulty. Both Perrett et al. (1982) and Baylis et al. (1985) included a variety of objects along with faces in their studies of neuronal selectivity in the temporal lobe, and did find occasional selectivity for certain nonface objects as well as for faces. However, they note that the maximal response obtained with faces was invariably stronger than the maximal response obtained with other objects. They concluded that these neurons respond preferentially to faces, but do not have absolute specificity for faces.

It should be noted that the foregoing studies might underestimate the role of temporal neurons in representing nonface objects such as animals, plants, makes of autombile, etc., for two reasons. First, lab-reared monkeys would not have the range of visual experience with these stimuli that a human or free-ranging monkey would have, although they would have visual experience with faces. Without knowing the relative contributions of innate structure and experience in setting up and tuning these temporal neurons, we cannot know how much the null result should be expected simply on the basis of these monkeys' limited visual experience. Second, the fact that the recognition impairment in prosopagnosia is more severe for faces than for other categories of stimuli (so much so that for decades it was thought to be confined to faces) should lead us to expect fewer cells and/or more broadly-tuned cells for responding to animals, foods, etc. This, in turn, predicts that such cells would be harder to discover. In sum, the single unit recording literature offers evidence that is directly relevant to the stimulus-specific recognition system hypothesis. The available data are supportive of this hypothesis, although more data on nonface objects are needed before this source of evidence can be considered conclusive.

There is also some evidence from human prosopagnosics relevant to the "stimulus-specific recognition systems" hypothesis. The studies of L.H. and M.B. discussed earlier support the hypothesis, as recognition of living things was disproportionately impaired even when several other factors determining recognition difficulty were accounted for, and visual imagery for living things was disproportionately impaired even when difficulty for normal subjects was accounted for.

There is one other source of indirect evidence that should also be noted before leaving the topic of stimulus-specific recognition systems. Stimulus-specificity has emerged in many computational vision systems because of computational constraints. Some of the most successful visual object recognition systems are designed to work in extremely circumscribed stimulus domains, for example, manufacturing parts (Ikeuchi, 1987) or aerial views of terrain (Herman and Kanade, 1986). More relevant to the present issue, attempts to build systems of general applicability have also achieved greater success with certain types of stimuli than with others. For example, Marr and Nishihara's (1978) use of generalized cylinders works well for representing a variety of animals, but poorly for representing faces. Lowe's (1987) model-based system for recognition of 3D objects from novel viewpoints works well for rigid objects, but not for nonrigid objects. This suggests that the problem of building a completely general-purpose recognition system might best be solved by building two or more subsystems with differing strengths and weaknesses, and thus provides some independent motivation for interpreting prosopagnosia as damage to a stimulus-specific subsystem.

If prosopagnosia is caused by damage to a stimulus-specific recognition system, the question then arises: What aspect of a visual stimulus determines whether it will be recognized using that special system? What is "special" about the class stimuli with which prosopagnosics have trouble? In at least one case (De Renzi, case 4) this class seems to

include only faces; in many other cases it includes stimuli that are living
or related to living things: faces, animals, plants, foods, clothing (as it is
tailored to the human form), as well as stimuli that are not even remotely
derived from "organic" forms: makes of automobile and buildings. One
could argue, not altogether implausibly, that the latter group of stimuli
may be recognized *as if* they were organic, that is, using a system that
originally evolved for the recognition of living things. Unfortunately,
there is no way to find out whether this is true or just a plausible story.
A more fruitful approach would be to consider what the *formal* characteristics of stimuli in this category might be. What kind of shape coding is
heavily demanded by faces, demanded to a lesser extent by animals,
plants, clothing, makes of automobile, and buildings, and still less by
other stimuli? One possible answer to this question is offered in section
5.5.

5.3 Pure Alexia

5.3.1 Disconnection accounts of pure alexia
The syndrome of pure alexia has been interpreted in three ways with
respect to models of normal visual recognition. The first is a disconnection account, originally proposed by Dejerine (1892) and more recently
championed by Geschwind (1965). According to this account, reading
consists of associating visual information in occipital cortex with language representations in posterior language areas. This was done by way
of the left angular gyrus, adjacent to Wernicke's area, which is hypothesized to contain stored multimodal associations linking the visual and
sound patterns of printed words. Thus, pure alexia results from any
lesion that disconnects the visual cortex from the left angular gyrus. The
neuropathology of pure alexia is generally consistent with this hypothesis (e.g., Damasio and Damasio, 1983; Greenblatt, 1983), often involving
a left occipital lesion (causing blindness in the right visual field) and
damage to the adjacent splenium (disconnecting left visual field information from the left hemisphere). Despite the anatomical support for this
interpretation of pure alexia, many of the problems with disconnection
accounts of object agnosia apply here as well. For example, why should
pure alexia be dissociable from object agnosia, prosopagnosia, optic
aphasia, and color naming deficits? In addition, although it is not in any
way *inconsistent* with the letter-by-letter reading stategy of pure alexic
patients, it is also not explanatory of this highly characteristic feature of
the syndrome. It is, of course, possible that disconnection may contribute
to some cases of pure alexia. That is, the effects of whatever mechanism
accounts for the selectivity of the alexic impairment for written material,

and forces the patient to use a letter-by-letter reading strategy may be exacerbated by superimposed disconnection between relevant brain areas.

5.3.2 Pure alexia as a material-specific agnosia

The general idea that pure alexia is a category-specific visual agnosia for verbal material, endorsed by many writers, was first cast in the form of a specific hypothesis by Warrington and Shallice (1980). According to them, normal fluent reading requires that the individually recognized letters be grouped into recognizable higher-order units, corresponding to morphemes and/or whole words. They term these higher-order visual representations "word forms" and hypothesize that pure alexic patients have sustained damage to the word form system. This explains why their ability to recognize words seems to be mediated solely by recognizing a single letter at a time.

The evidence presented by Warrington and Shallice for damaged word forms in pure alexia is of two kinds. First, they attempted to show that their pure alexic patients have good or at least adequate visual perception of letters and words, ruling out a visual perceptual locus for the impairment. The specific tests of visual perception that they used will be discussed below. By a process of elimination, they argue, this strengthens the support for a higher-order locus of impairment. Second, they showed that these patients had much more difficulty reading script than print. One characteristic of script writing is that the individual letters are less distinctive than individual printed characters, and therefore recognition of words in script relies more on overall word form than the recognition of printed words. Thus, the greater impairment with script is consistent with a word form deficit.

Patterson and Kay (1982) proposed a modification of the word form hypothesis, according to which the word form system is intact, but that its input from letter recognition systems is limited to one letter at a time. This hypothesis can account for all of Warrington and Shallice's data. In fact, both versions of the word form hypothesis are compatible with all of the data collected by Warrington and Shallice and Patterson and Kay, and both groups acknowledge this (Patterson and Kay, 1982; Shallice, 1987, chapter 4). Patterson and Kay's reasons for preferring their alternative include several indirect and, in their words, "intuitive" considerations. One of the most compelling is their observation that for some patients "enormous effort was required to identify letters; but, once that had been achieved, moving from letters to the word was virtually automatic" (p. 433). This is the opposite of what one would expect if the word forms themselves were damaged.

A recent study by Bub et al. (1989) presents striking evidence of the availability of word form information in a pure alexic patient. These authors carried out a "word superiority effect" experiment with their patient. Recall from section 3.3.1 that word superiority refers to the fact that individual letters in a letter string are perceived more quickly and clearly when the letter string is a word than when it is a nonword. This effect cannot be attributed to just guessing the identity of a letter based on the partial or full perceptions of the other letters in the word, because it can be demonstrated even in a forced choice task in which both of the letter choices make a word. For example, if the stimulus word is "cap," and the choices for the final letter are "p" and "t," subjects will be more successful at choosing "p," even though "t" would also make a word, than if the letter string had been "dat" and the same choice of final letters given. Bub et al. showed that a word superiority effect was present in the pure alexic patient that they tested, and that it was of roughly the same magnitude as that shown by an age-matched control subject with an equivalent visual field defect but no alexia. The ability of higher-order, multiletter patterns to affect the encoding of individual letters in a word demonstrates rather directly that such higher-order multiletter patterns are available in pure alexia. Thus, these results disconfirm the word form hypothesis of Warrington and Shallice, at least in the one case of Bub et al. They can be accommodated by Patterson and Kay's modified word form hypothesis, on the assumption that constraints from stored word form information can facilitate letter analysis even when letters gain access to the word form level one at a time.

5.3.3 Pure alexia as a manifestation of perceptual impairment

The third general approach to explaining pure alexia in terms of impairments in normal processing implicates visual perception as the locus of processing failure. Specifically, the hypothesis is that pure alexia is a manifestation of ventral simultanagnosia, the impairment in our normal ability to rapidly recognize multiple objects. Before considering the evidence for and against this hypothesis, let us consider a very general implication of the choice between it and the previous hypothesis.

The existence of a selective impairment for reading, without concomitant impairments in other visual or language processes, implies that there is some region of the brain that is necessary for *and dedicated to* reading. If either version of the word form hypothesis is true, this implies that localized brain functions include functions that are evolutionarily very recent, that require extensive instruction to learn, and that relatively few individuals in the history of the species have ever possessed. While not a priori impossible, this conclusion represents a surprising departure from the other functions that we know to be localized (perception, motor control, language, memory). Thus, the issue of whether pure alexia represents a selective impairment for reading per se, or whether it is a manifestation of a more general perceptual impairment, has implications beyond our understanding of reading impairments. It bears on the issue of how the functional architecture of the mind is mapped onto the physical architecture of the brain, and in particular on the distinction between the kinds of psychological processes that make use of localized, dedicated hardware and the kinds that do not.

Despite the far-reaching implications of the choice between viewing pure alexia as an agnosia specific to written material and as a more general visual impairment, there has been relatively little effort directed at distinguishing between these possibilities. Perhaps this is because the hypothesis of general visual impairment seems so unlikely on the face of things: After all, no gross visual disturbances are obvious on casual observation of these patients, and yet their reading disturbance is quite gross and obvious. The two best-known attempts to test the hypothesis, by Warrington and Shallice (1980) and Patterson and Kay (1982), rejected it based on the performance of their patients on various tests of visual perception. However, it is a neuropsychological truism that abilities such as visual perception are composed of many distinct and dissociable subprocesses, and it therefore follows that patients who pass certain tests of visual perception with flying colors could be severely impaired on others. Let us examine the tests of visual perception that Warrington, Shallice, Patterson and Kay administered to their patients, and consider whether these tests tapped the specific ability believed to be lacking in ventral simultanagnosic patients.

Warrington and Shallice (1980) carried out several different tests of visual perception with a mildly impaired case, R.A.V.: In Shallice's (1987, chapter 4) review of the different degrees of reading impairment in pure alexia, discussed in the last chapter, R.A.V. was the least impaired of eight cases. He required less than 2 seconds to read three- and four-letter words and only 3 seconds to read seven- and eight-letter words (the other seven cases reviewed by Shallice required on average 8.5 seconds and 21 seconds, respectively). On two standard tests of reading he scored well: On the Schonell graded word reading test he performed "at a high level" (98/100), and on the Nelson reading test he obtained a reading IQ of 121. Thus, his impairment was evident only in the slowness with which he read most text. Warrington and Shallice also administered a few of their visual tests to a second case, J.D.C., who was more impaired than R.A.V. Patterson and Kay (1982) replicated some of Warrington and Shallice's results with their case, T.P., whose severity is in the middle range of the cases reviewed by Shallice (1987, chapter 4).

Both Warrington and Shallice (1980) and Patterson and Kay (1982) assessed the effects of visual angle and number of distracting characters on their cases' ability to recognize alphanumeric characters. Displays such as "6STOP4" were shown tachistoscopically, with instructions to read the digits in the first and last position. For both Warrington and Shallice's case, R.A.V., and Patterson and Kay's case, T.P., performance was unaffected by the number of intervening letters. Similarly, R.A.V. was able to read the central letter in a tachistoscopic display of five letters, and his ability to read two briefly presented letters, while not perfect, was unaffected by how far apart they were spaced. Does this mean that these patients did not have an impairment in the rapid recognition of multiple characters? No, because these tasks did not require the recognition of the distractor characters, and the characters to be recognized were in positions known by the subject in advance. Levine and Calvanio (1978) demonstrated that ventral simultanagnosics are unaffected by distractor letters when the position of the letter to be reported was known in advance. Therefore, on the hypothesis that pure alexics suffer from ventral simultanagnosia, they would not be predicted to show detrimental effects of number of distracting letters in the tasks just described. Furthermore, Kinsbourne and Warrington (1962) demonstrated that spatial separation amongst the stimuli to be recognized has no effect on ease of recognition, again predicting that the separation manipulation would not affect the performance of R.A.V. and T.P even if they were simultanagnosics. In a different type of task, Warrington and Shallice gave R.A.V., and the more impaired J.D.C., an array of 25 letters to read aloud without time pressure. They report that R.A.V. completed the task flawlessly, and J.D.C. made only three errors; time to complete the task is not reported. As before, this finding is as consistent with the ventral simultanagosia hypothesis as with the hypothesis of no visual impairment: Kinsbourne and Warrington stressed the idea that simultanagnosia is a disorder of *rapid* visual encoding, and that given sufficient time a simultanagnosic could recognize arbitrarily many stimuli.

Warrington and Shallice also present the results of three tachistoscopic "whole report" tasks with R.A.V. When shown 3 letters simultaneously for 50 ms (unmasked), R.A.V. made only 8 errors out of 40 trials. When shown 4 digits simultaneously for 100 ms (unmasked), R.A.V. made 5 errors out of 20 trials. Finally, when shown strings of 5 letters that were either randomly chosen or statistical approximations to English for 100 ms (unmasked), R.A.V. reported 53 percent of the random letters and 72 percent of the letters in strings approximating English. Although these levels of performance are above those of the simultanagnosics studied by Kinsbourne and Warrington (1962) and Levine and Calvanio (1978), R.A.V. is an extremely mild alexic and would therefore be expected to show only mild simultanagnosia. Furthermore, the absence of control data makes it difficult to determine whether these findings confirm or disconfirm the hypothesis that R.A.V. is a mild simultanagnosic. Although Warrington and Shallice point out that his performance is roughly equivalent to the mean performance of left-hemisphere-damaged patients tested in the same task by Warrington and Rabin (1971), the latter patients viewed the stimuli for less time (50 ms), which would make the task harder.

Finally, Warrington and Shallice cite the good performance of their patients on various clinical tests involving picture interpretation as evidence against simultanagnosia. Their patients were tested with the Peabody picture vocabulary test, the WAIS picture completion test, and the WAIS picture arrangement test. Although J.D.C. performed well below average on all three of these tests, R.A.V. performed well, rating "high average range" on the two WAIS subtests. Once again, these tests are not the appropriate ones for detecting simultanagnosia: With the exception of picture arrangement, which involves sequencing simple scenes, they do not require that multiple objects be recognized in relation to one another, as is the case with the pictures traditionally used to detect simultanagosia, such as the Binet-Bobertag picture or the "telegraph boy" picture (see figure 5) used by Kinsbourne and Warrington (1962). Given the mildness of R.A.V.'s reading deficit, and the lack of emphasis on speed in the one relevant test, the picture arrangement test (1–2 minutes are normally allowed for performing each item, Wechsler, 1981), success on this test is not strong evidence against simultanagnosia. One might as easily conclude from his high performance on the unspeeded reading tests mentioned earlier that he is not alexic! The appropriate test of visual recognition of nonverbal material would parallel their tests with verbal material with this patient, that is, it would be carried out tachistoscopically.

Friedman and Alexander (1984) performed such a contrast, between the recognition of tachistoscopically presented verbal and nonverbal visual material, with a pure alexic patient. When the tasks involved simple stimulus detection, discriminating the orientation of lines presented individually, or recognizing which of two letters was presented individually, the pure alexic's thresholds were within the range of the normal subjects'. In contrast, when the task involved recognizing words or line drawings, the pure alexic's thresholds were elevated, to an equal extent, with respect to the normal subjects' thresholds. Friedman and Alexander conclude that "pure alexia is the behavioral manifestation of a deficit in the speed of visual identification, which is not specific to orthographic material" (p. 9).[1]

Another argument against an early perceptual locus for the impairment in pure alexia comes from Bub et al. (1989). They suggest that their finding of a word superiority effect is inconsistent with the hypothesis that pure alexia is a manifestation of ventral simultanagnosia. They state that, in contrast to the claims of Kinsbourne and Warrington (1962) and Levine and Calvanio (1978) regarding the association between simultanagnosia and pure alexia, "the nature of J.V.'s responding on words and pseudowords [compared to nonwords in the word superiority experiment] implies that his perceptual deficit must affect the retrieval of multiple letters *after* they have been identified" (p. 366). These authors appear to be assuming that the top-down influences of orthographic context in the word superiority effect do not affect the actual visual perception and recognition of individual letters. However, this assumption is incorrect: There is a large literature in cognitive psychology demonstrating that the word superiority effect alters visual recognition of words *at the letter level* (McClelland and Rumelhart, 1981). Therefore, the Bub et al. findings are consistent with the hypothesis that pure alexia is a manifestation of ventral simultanagnosia. So far we have reviewed evidence that was initially taken to disprove the hypothesis that pure alexia results from a visual impairment, and shown that this evidence does not disprove the hypothesis. However, the evidence so far reviewed does not prove the hypothesis either. What would constitute strong evidence for the hypothesis that pure alexia is just ventral simultanagnosia—that is, that the two impairments have been studied in different contexts and labelled with different names, but are actually the same impairment? One would have to test a large number of pure alexic patients and ventral simultanagnosic patients and find that in each case both impairments were present. Although such a research project has yet to be carried out, we can review what is known about the simultaneous form perception of pure alexics and the reading of ventral simultanagnosics and see whether any of these opportunities for disconfirming the hypothesis in fact do so.

Most pure alexics misperceive letters while reading. This is not predicted by the word form hypothesis, but is what one would expect if patients are simultanagnosic. Patterson and Kay (1982) examined the nature of the errors made by four pure alexic patients and found that they were strongly dependent on visual similarity. Figure 26 is a confusion matrix, showing which letters were mistaken for which other letters. Because the letters on the axes are ordered in such a way that similar-looking letters are adjacent to one another, the clustering of errors near the main diagonal indicates the influence of visual similarity on pure alexics' letter identification errors. This is what one would expect if visual

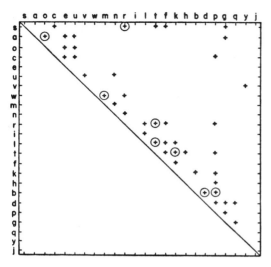

Figure 26
A confusion matrix for lowercase letters, based on errors made by Patterson and Kay's (1980) pure alexic patients. Visually similar letters are close together in the ordering. Confusions that occurred only a few times or less are marked with the symbol +; those that occurred more often are marked with the + inside a circle.

perception were at fault in these patients and is consistent with the observations of Levine and Calvanio (1978) of their simultanagnosic patients, who also made predominantly visual errors.

Bub et al. (1989) administered a letter-matching task to their pure alexic patient, in which he was to decide whether a pair of simultaneously presented letters were identical or not. Normal subjects perform this task more quickly if they are first shown one of the letters in the letter pair before the presentation of the letter pair (e.g., an "A" coming before either an "AA" or an "AB") and more slowly if they are first shown an irrelevant letter. The pure alexic did not show this pattern of performance. Instead, he was not significantly faster when shown a matching letter first and was disproportionately slowed down by the occurrence of an irrelevant letter. In the words of Bub et al. "the mere presence of a letter before the onset of another letter pair inhibits their analysis" (p. 374). Recall from chapter 2 that Kinsbourne and Warrington (1962) found the same thing with their simultanagnosic patients: Sequentially presented letters contributed to the simultanagnosic "bottleneck" in recognition as much as simultaneously presented letters.

In evaluating the hypothesis that pure alexia and ventral simultanagnosia are the same, we should assess the reading ability of ventral simultanagnosics as well as the simultaneous form perception abilities of pure alexics. In the two small group studies described earlier by Kinsbourne and Warrington (1962) and Levine and Calvanio (1978), the patients were all alexic. It is difficult to interpret the results of the large group study reported by Warrington and Rabin (1971), as the authors give only group averages. Without knowing how many individual patients in the left posterior group were impaired in the perception task, and how many of these patients had reading difficulties, we cannot assess the strength of relation between alexia and simultanagnosia.

Although decisive evidence is lacking, the available evidence is certainly consistent with the hypothesis that pure alexia is a manifestation of ventral simultanagnosia. Any stimuli that tax patients' ability to rapidly identify multiple forms will be difficult for these patients to recognize. Printed words are the prime example of such stimuli and, outside of laboratories with tachistoscopes, reading will be the only activity where these patients will have pronounced recognition deficits. A very general implication of this hypothesis is that we need not postulate a neurological "module" for the specific acquired skill of reading.

This interpretation of pure alexia could be taken to imply that the syndrome is an "apperceptive" rather than an "associative" agnosia. To some extent, the distinction between these two general types of agnosia is academic: As already argued in the cases of associative agnosia in general and prosopagnosia in particular, all of the agnosias seem attributable to faulty perception. The more relevant distinction concerns the level of visual processing at which perception is impaired. In the case of associative object agnosia and prosopagnosia, as well as pure alexia or ventral simultanagnosia, the perceptual impairment does seem to occur at a higher level than the other agnosias traditionally classified as "apperceptive": Stimuli are detected even if they are not all recognized immediately, in contrast to dorsal simultanagnosia, and problems with low-level perceptual grouping of contour segments into a perceived whole do not appear to be present, in contrast to the narrow sense of the category of apperceptive agnosia.

5.4 Other Category-specific Deficits

5.4.1 Semantic versus formal categories and the organization of visual recognition

The evidence reviewed in the previous two sections on the question of category specificity in prosopagnosia and pure alexia could be summarized as answering the question with a "well, yes and no." That is, there is evidence of relatively selective impairment in these syndromes, such that the recognition of certain kinds of stimuli is more impaired than the recognition of other kinds of stimuli. However, the sets of impaired and spared stimuli do not constitute "categories" in the sense of *semantic* categories such as "faces," "living things," or "verbal material." Rather, it seems likely that they are determined by structural or *formal* visual properties, such as the number of separate parts that must be recognized in order to recognize the whole.

Even Konorski's (1967) nine different "gnostic fields," shown in figure 19, have a formal basis in his taxonomy. Although his interpretation is speculative, and the nine dissociable categories themselves come largely from anecdotal observations, he provides a good illustration of the way in which apparently semantic distinctions can be accounted for in terms of relatively simple formal distinctions, such as the kinds of shape primitives that could be used, variations in viewing conditions, relations with perceptual information in other modalities. For example, he accounts for the putative dissociation between common objects on the one hand and landmark objects such as buildings and trees on the other in this way: "(1) Small manipulable objects or everyday living. The common feature of these objects are (a) they have sharply defined contours . . . (b) they are moveable—that is, they are not associated with a given background, (c) they are seen not only from varying distances . . . but from different sides . . . [Larger, partially manipulable objects:] A separate group of stimulus objects probably belonging to the same category is composed of larger objects which can neither be visually perceived at one glance (unless from a distance), nor handled as a whole . . . (2) Nonmanipulable objects perceived only by vision . . . usually unmovable and are closely related to the stimulus background against which they are seen . . . Another characteristic feature of these objects is that they are strongly related to the vertical axis of our visual field" (p. 118). The evidence reviewed in the last chapter suggests that the only neuropsychological phenomena that involve semantically based selective deficits are outside of the realm of visual recognition per se, in parts of the cognitive system that may be engaged by visual tasks, but are also engaged by nonvisual, purely verbal tasks.

What does the absence of specifically semantic dissociations in visual recognition impairments tell us about the normal operation of visual recognition? To answer this question, it would be helpful first to consider the more general question of how the presence or absence of any kind of category-specific recognition impairment, semantic or formal, can be interpreted. If we view object recognition as the recovery of a unique representation of an object's true shape from the multitude of different images that the object can cast on the retina under different viewing conditions, then any kind of invariances among the different images of a particular object will help us to recognize the object. Konorski's account of his various "gnostic fields" makes explicit the fact that different kinds of stimuli have different kinds of invariances: Some will always have sharp contours, some are always seen in one particular orientation, some are always seen against the same background, some are rigid, and so on. To the extent that different categories of stimuli have different invariances, recognition of these stimuli can be made more efficient by processing stimuli differently (i.e., processing different aspects of them). Damage to one of these specialized forms of processing would then cause a category-specific recognition impairment. The existence of such impairments is therefore consistent with the hypothesis that the visual system has evolved special-purpose recognition subsystems that exploit the different kinds of invariances available in different stimulus domains.

In this context, the question of whether or not there are category-specific recognition impairments for *semantic* categories is related to the question of whether the semantic identity of an object contributes constraints that could be exploited in recognizing the object more efficiently. Do objects from particular semantic categories have characteristic invariances that relate their retinal images to their true shape? In principle, there may be some very indirect and weak regularities (if not *invariances*) associated with different images from particular semantic categories. In fact, early artificial intelligence vision systems exploited such regularities in parsing and identifying objects in scenes differently, depending upon the semantic nature of the scene. For example, the vision system of Tenenbaum and Barrow (1976, cited in Marr, 1982) used knowledge about locales such as offices to recognize the objects in an office scene. Knowing that desks generally have phones on them, the system would be more likely to identify a black blob halfway up the image as a phone. In such a system, it would be possible to have "office agnosia," that is, impaired ability to recognize just office objects following damage to the system's knowledge about offices. The absence of cases of visual agnosia for semantically-based categories of stimuli suggests that our visual systems do not work this way. Whatever regularities might exist amongst the different images of stimuli from common semantic categories, our visual system has not developed specialized subsystems to exploit them.

5.4.2 Narrow versus broad categories and the implementation of visual representation
Another difference between the category-specific deficits that are attributable to impairments in visual recognition per se and those attributable to other parts of the cognitive system is the breadth of the categories. The

categories of impairment in visual recognition deficits are broad: In prosopagnosia the impairment encompasses some subset of faces, animals, plants, buildings, clothing, and makes of automobile, and in pure alexia it encompasses all stimuli for which rapid identification of multiple parts or objects is required. In contrast, the categories of impairment in naming deficits can be quite narrow (for example, body parts or fruits and vegetables). Why should this be the case? What determines the breadth of categories that can be selectively impaired?

A strong constraint on the breadth of selective impairments comes from the nature of the representations themselves and their neural instantiation. In particular, the degree to which a representation is *local* or *distributed* will strongly constrain the breadth of the impairment. Let us consider the computational properties of local and distributed representations that are relevant to understanding selective losses of visual and semantic knowledge after brain damage.

In systems that use local representation, there is a neuron or set of neurons dedicated to representing one entity (item, category, or whatever). This is equivalent to the "grandmother cell" theory of representation. For example, daffodils might be represented by one neuron or set of neurons, and roses by a different and disjoint set. In local representations, there is a one-to-one correspondence between the things being represented and the neurons instantiating their representation: Each entity is represented by a different neuron or set of neurons, and each neuron or set of neurons represents one entity.

In contrast, distributed representations use the same set of neurons to represent different entities, and the representation of a given entity is said to be "distributed" over the set of neurons. How are distributed representations distinguishable, if the same set of neurons is used to represent more than one entity? By the *pattern* of levels of activity over the different neurons. Roses might correspond to a certain subset of neurons being highly activated, others being moderately activated, and a third subset being inactive. Daffodils would also be represented by various levels of activation over this same set of neurons, but not the same pattern as for roses; perhaps some of the neurons that were highly activated for roses would be only moderately active or downright inactive when representing daffodils, whereas other neurons might be more active when representing daffodils than roses. In sum, for distributed representations each entity is represented by a pattern of activity over many neurons, and these neurons are involved in representing many different entities.

Having set up the dichotomy between local and distributed representations, it should be noted that there are degrees of distributedness. A system can represent all entities using different patterns of activation over all of its neurons, which would be a form of maximally distributed representation, or it could represent certain sets of stimuli by patterns of activation over certain sets of neurons. It is clear that the brain does not use maximally distributed representations: Occipital neurons are not involved in representing sounds, for example. More likely, there are sets of stimuli (delineated by modality, for example) that are represented in a distributed manner by sets of neurons. Hinton et al. (1986) put it thus: "The representations advocated here are local at a global scale but global [i.e., distributed] at a local scale" (p. 79).

Another qualification on the idea of distributed representation is that a given pattern of activation over a given set of units will be a distributed representation of some things and a local representation of others. In the example of a distributed representation of a rose, the individual units that are activated each represent some "microfeature" (as Hinton et al., 1986, put it) of the rose in a local manner. These microfeatures might correspond to the kinds of English-language features that we would attribute to a rose, such as redness, smelling sweet, having thorns, and so on, or they might correspond to some other, less intuitive predicates that can be used to represent a rose and that are shared to varying degrees with other things being represented in the same set of units.

The distributed nature of representations, within a particular processing domain at least, is consistent with most of what neuropsychology tells us about neural representation. For example, an important property of distributed representations, which they seem to share with real neural representations, is their "graceful" or hologram-style degradation after damage. Because no representation depends upon just one small set of neurons, then small amounts of damage to the system will never wipe out any particular representation. This is in contrast to current computers, in which the removal of one part of the memory representing a program could cause the entire system to crash (a difference that has been used to argue that the brain cannot be a computer, when it really only implies that the brain's computations are carried out on distributed rather than local representations). A small amount of local damage will cause the large number of representations that depend *partly* on the damaged subset of neurons to be degraded just a bit. This is consistent with the apparent robustness of the brain to most small lesions.

An apparent discrepancy between the idea of distributed representations and empirical findings from neuroscience involves the single unit recordings discussed in section 5.2.2. Doesn't the existence of face-selective neurons, including neurons selective for particular faces, imply that the visual system uses extremely local representations for face recognition? No, because although these cells respond more to one face than another, there is a range of faces to which they will respond, and conversely, a given face will evoke responses of varying degrees in a large number of neurons. In other words, within the domain of face representation at least, the results of single unit recordings imply that distributed representations are being used.

It is apparent from what has already been said about local versus distributed representations that selective losses of knowledge can only be as narrow as the knowledge representations are local. That is, if a particular domain of knowledge, such as the visual appearances of faces, is represented in a distributed manner, then selective losses within that domain will be impossible: Any damage that one does to any *part* of the system will affect knowledge of *all* of the entities being represented by that part of the system, and in distributed representations all entities are represented using all parts of the system. Given that selective disorders of object recognition are relatively broad compared to disorders of naming, this would imply that visual knowledge is represented in a more distributed manner than the knowledge underlying naming.

Why would the knowledge underlying naming be represented relatively locally, allowing for selective loss of knowledge specific to categories as narrow as fruits and vegetables, compared to the knowledge underlying visual recognition, which seems to be more distributed? In order to answer this question, one last property of distributed representations must be pointed out. Representations of similar things will generally consist of similar patterns of activation in the network. This is because they will share similar sets of microfeatures. For most purposes, this is an excellent property for a system of representations to have. It allows the system to generalize knowledge about one entity automatically to other similar entities. If the system learns that roses need water, then it will tend to generalize this knowledge to daffodils. Within the domain of visual object recognition, this is probably useful more often than not, as similar-looking images are likely to result from either the very same object or objects with similar properties. In other words, similar-looking images are associated with objects that should be treated similarly. This is because there is a nonarbitrary relation between the appearance of an object and other knowledge that one might access about the object in the process of visual recognition. In contrast, similar-sounding words are not generally associated with objects that should be treated similarly. It is the very arbitrariness of the relations between words and their referents that makes language a prime example of a symbol system. For this reason, the automatic generalization of distributed representations is a disadvantage for naming operations, and we might expect that the brain has evolved more local forms of representation to subserve naming. This is consistent with the observation that the only superselective category-specific impairments reviewed earlier are related to naming.

5.5 Two Kinds of Associative Agnosia?

Patterns of association and dissociation among abilities after brain damage are often used to make inferences about the organization of cognitive processes underlying those abilities. Within certain boundary conditions (see Shallice, 1988, chapter 10), a dissociation between two abilities implies that they rely on different components of the functional architecture of the mind. A reliable association between abilities is consistent with the hypothesis that they rely on common internal processes, although it is also consistent with neuroanatomic proximity of functionally distinct processes, such that lesions affecting one process will affect the other. What do the patterns of covariation among different forms of associative agnosia suggest about the functional architecture of visual object recognition?

One theoretically tantalizing dissociation within the associative agnosias is between face recognition and the recognition of other kinds of objects. As discussed in chapter 4, there are cases of prosopagnosia in which the recognition of objects other than faces is only mildly, if at all, affected. There are also cases in which the recognition of certain objects other than faces is obviously disturbed, most often animals, plants, buildings, makes of automobile, etc. Even in these cases, the patients' preserved ability to recognize a variety of other objects makes it inappropriate to categorize them as across-the-board associative object agnosics. The opposite dissociation, impaired object recognition with roughly intact face recognition, has also been observed.

A second double dissociation has been observed between the recognition of printed words and other objects. There are a number of associative agnosic patients who have no obvious problems recognizing printed words. In addition, the vast majority of patients with pure alexia are not agnosic for objects.

The pairwise dissociability of both face and written word recognition from object recognition might seem to imply that there are three corresponding types of visual recognition ability. However, this three-part organization for visual recognition would follow only if all possible *triads* of spared and impaired recognition of faces, objects, and words were observed to occur. Based on a review of the literature (Farah, in press), there are certain combinations of these abilities that are not observed, and it is possible to account for the patterns that do occur with only two hypothesized components of recognition. What these two components might consist of is most easily described by first introducing the idea of a "structural description."

A structural description is a very general term referring to visual representations of shape that are composed of parts and the spatial relations among the parts. The parts may be relatively simple or complex enough to be considered objects in their own right. Most cognitive psychologists and computer scientists studying vision favor some form or other of structural description for the representations of shape underlying object recognition (Pinker, 1985). Of course, this still leaves open a wide range of possible representations, and an important goal in vision research is therefore to specify more precisely the nature of the parts and relations.

Even without knowing what kinds of parts the visual system uses in decomposing shapes, it is probably correct to assume that some objects will be decomposed into more parts, and hence more elementary parts, than others. Some objects may not be decomposed at all, but recognized as a single unit, all of a piece. If we assume that our ability to know whether a single part has come from a particular object is roughly indicative of whether that part is explicitly represented in our structural description of the object, then we can hazard some guesses about which objects are recognized via decomposition into simpler parts and which are recognized with little or no decomposition. Face recognition seems to be a likely candidate for the latter type of process. We are not apt to know whether an isolated facial feature came from a particular face or not: We could know Jim's face very well but not be able to say whether or not a fragment of a photograph showing only the nose was from a photograph of Jim. The fact that most face-selective cells in the primate visual system respond to whole faces and do not respond to individual components presented in isolation, nor to the full set of features presented in an altered spatial arrangement, is also supportive of the idea that faces are recognized "all of a piece" rather than by decomposition into simpler parts. To a lesser extent, it is difficult to know whether an ear or a tail viewed in isolation came from a particular animal; a cat's ear looks much like a horse's ear. In contrast, we can often make accurate guesses about the sources of other relatively simple object parts: a key from a typewriter keyboard, a doorknob, the sharpened end of a pencil lead. This is consistent with the idea that our representations of these objects include these parts, explicitly represented as parts. Printed words are the clearest case of objects that are decomposed into simpler part units: There is no doubt whether the letter "c" does or doesn't come from the word "cat."

Among the many abilities that we must possess if we do indeed represent objects using structural descriptions are the following: First, the ability to represent the parts themselves, including quite complex parts for objects that undergo little or no shape decomposition. (For an object such as a face, which by hypothesis undergoes little or no decomposition, the "part" may be the whole object.) Second, the ability to rapidly encode multiple parts, especially for objects that undergo decomposition into many parts. These two abilities suggest an interpretation for the two components of visual recognition that were inferred from the patterns of cooccurrence among impairments in face, object and word recognition. The conjecture being offered here is that impairments in these two abilities underlie the range of associative agnosic phenomena. In other words, associative agnosia can be understood in terms of difficulty encoding complex parts or difficulty encoding numerous parts, or some combination of the two.

On this account, if the representation of parts is only mildly impaired, then most objects will be recognized, and only those objects that undergo little or no decomposition into parts, and whose parts are therefore relatively complex, will be affected. This corresponds to prosopagnosia. If the representation of parts is more severely impaired, then the recognition deficit will extend to more objects, and only objects with the simplest parts will be recognized. This corresponds to object agnosia with prosopagnosia but without alexia. If the ability to represent parts is intact, but the ability to rapidly encode multiple parts is impaired, then most objects will be recognized. The only objects that will be affected will be those that undergo decomposition into many parts, and for which multiple parts must be encoded before recognition can occur. This corresponds to alexia. If the impairment in this ability is severe enough such that even a moderate number of parts cannot be rapidly and accurately encoded, then the recognition of objects other than words will be affected as well. However, even in this case faces should not be affected, as they do not require encoding multiple separate parts. This corresponds to agnosia with both alexia but without prosopagnosia. If both abilities are impaired, then the recognition of all objects will be affected. This corresponds to agnosia with both alexia and prosopagnosia.

This account places two constraints on the patterns of cooccurrence among the associative agnosias: First, that there can never be a case of object agnosia without either prosopagnosia or alexia. Second, that there can never be a case of prosopagnosia and alexia that does not also have *some* degree of object agnosia. Table 1 shows a set of 99 case reports that was used to test these predictions. The table is comprised of all adult cases of associative visual agnosia reported in English or French since 1966 listed in the "Medline" periodical data base, along with assorted

Table 1
Cases of associative agnosia, showing lesion localization and ability to recognize real or depicted faces, objects, and printed words.

Case	Lesion localization	Faces	Objects	Words
Aimard et al. (1981) #4	R temp	x		?
Albert et al. (1975)	Bilat temp-occ	x	x	
Aptman et al. (1977)[1]	Bilat occip	x	x	x
Assal (1969)	R par-occ	x		
Assal et al. (1984)	Bilat temp-occ	x		
Bauer (1982); see also Bauer and Trobe, (1984); Bauer, (1984)	Bilat temp-occ	x	x	
Bauer and Verfaellie (1988)	Bilat temp-occ	x	x	x
Benke (1988)	L par-occ	x	x	x
Benton and Van Allen (1972)	?	x	?	
Beyn and Knyazeva (1962)	Bilat occ	x	x	?
Bornstein and Kidron (1959)[2]	R par-occ	x		
Bornstein et al. (1969)	R posterior	x	?	
Boudouresques et al. (1972)	L occip	?	x	x
Boudouresques et al. (1979)	R temp-par	x	x	
Bruyer et al. (1983)	Bilat occip	x		
Cambier et al. (1980)	Bilat temp-occ	x	x	x
Cohn et al. (1974); Cohn et al. (1977)	Bilat temp-occ	x		
Cole and Perez-Cruet (1964)	?	x	x	
Damasio et al. (1982) #1	Bilat temp-occ	x	x	
Damasio et al. (1982) #2	Bilat temp-occ	x	x	x
Damasio et al. (1982) #3[3]	Bilat temp-occ	x		x
Davidoff and Wilson (1985)	?	x	x	x
De Haan et al. (1987); Young and De Haan (1988)	?	x	x	
De Renzi (1986) #1	R temp-occ	x	?	?
De Renzi (1986) #2	R temp-occ	x	?	?
Duara et al. (1975)	Bilat occip	x	x	
Dumont et al. (1981)[4]	L temp-occ; R par-occ		x	x
Feinberg et al. (1986)	L temp-occ		x	x
Gallois et al. (1988)[5]	L occip		x	x
Gloning et al. (1970)	Bilat temp-occ	x		
Gloning et al. (1970) appendix	?	x	x	x
Glowic and Violon (1981)	Bilat temp-occ	x		

Table 1 (continued)

Case	Lesion localization	Faces	Objects	Words
Gomori and Hawryluk (1984)	Bilat temp-occ	x	x	
Guard et al. (1981) [6]	L temp-occ; R temp	x	x	x
Hecaen and Ajuriaguerra (1956)	Left occip		x	x
Hecaen et al. (1974)[7]	Left occip		x	x
Karpov et al. (1979) #1	Bilat occip	x	x	x
Karpov et al. (1979) #2	R occip	x	x	x
Karpov et al. (1979) #3	L occip		x	x
Karpov et al. (1979) #4	L occip		x	x
Karpov et al. (1979) #5[8]	Bilat occip		x	
Kawahata and Nagata (1989)	Bilat temp-occ	x	x	x
Kay and Levin (1982) #1	Bilat temp-occ; R par	x		
Kay and Levin (1982) #2	Bilat occip	x		
Kay and Levin (1982) #3	R posterior	x		?
Kumar et al. (1986) #1	R temp-occ	x		
Kumar et al. (1986) #2	R temp-occ	x		?
Landis et al. (1986) #1	R temp-occ	x		
Landis et al. (1986) #2	R temp-occ	x	?	
Landis et al. (1986) #3	R temp-occ	x	?	?
Landis et al. (1986) #4	R par-occ	x	?	
Landis et al. (1986) #5	R par-temp-occ	x	?	
Landis et al. (1986) #6	R par-occ	x		?
Landis et al. (1988)	L par-occ; R temp-occ; R frontal	x	x	
Larrabee et al. (1985) #1[9]	L occip; R frontal	x	x	
Levin and Peters (1976)	?	x	?	
Levine (1978)	Right occip	x	x	
Levine and Calvanio (1989)	Bilat temp-occ; R front	x	x	
Lhermitte et al. (1969) #1	L temp-occ; R temp	x	x	x
Lhermitte et al. (1972)	L temp; R temp-occ	x	x	x
Lhermitte et al. (1973)[10]	L posterior	x	x	x
Lhermitte and Pillon (1975)	R temp-occ	x		
Mack and Boller (1977)	L par-occ; R occ	x	x	

Table 1 (continued)

Case	Lesion localization	Faces	Objects	Words
Macrae and Trolle (1956)	Bilat	x	x	x
Malone et al. (1982) #2	Bilat par-occ	x		
Marks and De Vito (1987) #1	Bilat temp-occ	x	x	x
Marks and De Vito (1987) #2[11]	R temp-par-occ		x	x
Marx et al. (1970)	Bilat posterior	x		
McCarthy and Warrington (1986)	L temp-occ		x	x
Mendez (1988) #1	?		x	x
Mendez (1988) #2	Bilat occip		x	x
Michel et al. (1986)	R temp-occ	x		
Nardelli et al. (1982) #1	Bilat temp-occ	x		
Nardelli et al. (1982) #2	Bilat temp-occ	x	x	?
Nardelli et al. (1982) #3	Bilat temp-occ	x		
Nardelli et al. (1982) #4	Bilat occ	x		
Newcombe and Ratcliff (1974) #1	?	x	x	
Newcombe and Ratcliff (1974) #2; Ratcliff and Newcombe (1982)	Bilat par-temp-occ	x	x	
Noel and Meyers (1971) #1	Bilat par-occ		x	x
Noel and Meyers (1971) #2	L posterior		x	x
Orgogozo et al. (1979) #2	L occip		x	x
Pallis (1955)	Bilat occip	x		
Pillon et al. (1981)[12]	L temp-par-occ		x	x
Raizada and Raizada (1972)	?	?	x	?
Renault et al. (1989)	R temp-occ	x		?
Riddoch and Humphreys (1987); Humpreys and Riddoch (1987a)	Bilat temp-occ	x	x	x
Rondot et al. (1967)	Bilat temp-occ	x		
Rubens and Benson (1971); Benson et al. (1973)	Bilat temp-occ	x	x	x
Shuttleworth et al. (1982) #1	Bilat temp-occ	x	x	x
Shuttleworth et al. (1982) #2	R temp-occ; L posterior	x	x	x
Striano et al. (1981)	Bilat temp-par-occ	x	x	
Taylor and Warrington (1971)	?	x	x	x
Tranel and Damasio (1988) #1; Tranel et al. (1988)	Bilat temp-occ	x		
Tranel and Damasio (1988) #2; Tranel et al. (1988)	Bilat occip	x		
Tranel and Damasio (1988) #3;	L temp;	x		

Table 1 (continued)

Case	Lesion localization	Faces	Objects	Words
Tranel et al. (1988)	R temp-occ			
Tzavaras et al. (1973)[13]	L temp	x		
Whitely and Warrington (1977) #1	Bilat occip	x		
Whitely and Warrington (1977) #2	R occip	x		
Whitely and Warrington (1977) #3	R occip	x		

A question mark in the localization column denotes either an absence of localizing information, or diffuse, nonlocalized damage. An "x" in the faces, objects or words column means that recognition of that category of visual stimulus was impaired; a question mark means that information concerning recognition of that category of stimulus was not given; and a blank means that recognition of that category of stimulus was tested and reported to be normal.
1. Patient was left-handed.
2. Possibility of bilateral damage noted.
3. Patient was termed prosopagnosic and alexic, but authors note recognition difficulties with cars and articles of clothing.
4. Right parietal-occipital lesion old and asymptomatic. Report mentions "prosopagnosia," but face recognition problems are exclusively anterograde and secondary to amnesia.
5. Patient was described as agnosic for objects and anomic for faces (i.e., not prosopagnosic).
6, 7. Some signs of optic aphasia superimposed on associative agnosia.
8. The two references to this case in the text of the article refer to him as nonagnosic; however, the table of cases lists a "slight object agnosia" among his neurological characteristics.
9. Three months postonset, when she was classified as "associative."
10. Authors remark that face recognition least affected.
11. Patient was ambidextrous.
12. Some signs of optic aphasia superimposed on associative agnosia.
13. Patient was left-handed.

cases from earlier articles and from book chapters.[2] Most of these cases include information about recognition of real or depicted faces, objects, and printed words, and this information is also listed in table 1, along with a brief description of lesion localization. Cases of pure alexia without any other agnosic features are too numerous to list and are not relevant to testing the hypothesis, as they do not have the potential to disconfirm it.

Of the 99 cases listed in table 1, there are only two occurrences of disconfirmatory patterns, and in both cases there is some inconsistency in the way these cases are described such that one description conforms to the predicted pattern and the other violates it. Case 5 of Karpov, Meerson and Tonkonough (1979) is described in their table of cases as having a "slight object agnosia" with no prosopagnosia or alexia. However, this case was also referred to twice in the text of the article as nonagnosic. Case 3 of Damasio et al. (1982) was described by the authors as prospagnosic and alexic, with no other neuropsychological impairments. However, case 3 is also described as handicapped in everyday life by his inability to recognize items such as clothing and cars, suggesting that there was some degree of object agnosia. Of the remaining 97 cases, none fails to conform to one of the five predicted patterns. In 9 of these, missing information has the potential to disconfirm the present account. For example, the brief report of Raizada and Raizada (1972) mentions object agnosia but gives no information about the patient's reading and face recognition abilities. If it were the case that both of these were intact, then the present account would be disconfirmed.

The neuropathology in these cases is also at least weakly supportive of the division being proposed here. Prosopagnosia generally follows bilateral lesions, although some nonautopsied cases appear to have unilateral right hemisphere lesions. Given that agnosia without alexia is interpreted as a more severe case of the same impairment that underlies prosopagnosia, then patients with agnosia without alexia should have have either bilateral or unilateral right lesions. Of the 15 cases reviewed here, 3 lacked localizing information, 2 had unilateral right hemisphere lesions affecting the visual areas of the brain, and 10 had bilateral lesions affecting the visual areas of the brain, mostly affecting the temporo-occipital regions. Two additional cases may be relevant as there were reported to be face and object recognition problems and no mention of reading problems. One patient had bilateral temporo-occipital lesions (Nardelli et al., 1982, case 2) and one had bilateral occipital lesions (Beyn and Knyazeva, 1962).

Given that pure alexia follows left posterior lesions, and that agnosia without prosopagnosia is interpreted as a more severe case of the same impairment that underlies pure alexia, it is then to be expected that cases of object agnosia without prosopagnosia would have left hemisphere lesions. Of the 16 cases reviewed here, one lacked localizing information, 10 had unilateral left hemisphere lesions affecting the visual areas of the brain (occipital lobe and neighboring parts of the temporal and parietal lobe), one had a unilateral right temporo-occipital lesion, and 4 had bilateral lesions. The case of unilateral right hemisphere damage was ambidextrous and had a left-handed brother (Marks and De Vito, 1987, case 2). One of the bilateral cases involved an old, asymptomatic right hemisphere lesion in the parieto-occipital area (Dumont et al., 1981). In another bilateral case (Larrabee et al., 1985) the right hemisphere lesion was in the frontal lobe, and hence unlikely to be related to the patient's visual recognition difficulties. A seventeenth case may also be relevant, as there were reading and object recognition difficulties noted with no mention of face recognition difficulties (Boudouresques et al., 1972); this patient had a left occipital lesion.

Finally, given the lesion sites associated with prosopagnosia and alexia, cases of across-the-board agnosia would be expected to have bilateral damage. Of the 22 cases of impaired face, object, and word recognition, 3 lacked localizing information, 16 had bilateral lesions affecting the visual areas of the brain (mostly temporo-occipital), one had a unilateral right posterior lesion, and 2 had unilateral left posterior lesions.

The interpretation of the two kinds of agnosia in terms of structural descriptions is admittedly speculative. There are other ways that the distinction between prosopagnosia and pure alexia has been expressed, which could also be applied to the distinction between agnosia without alexia and agnosia without prosopagnosia, respectively. Young (1988) relates word recognition to left hemisphere visual recognition processes, and face recognition to right hemisphere visual recognition processes. Levine and Calvanio (1989) distinguish between agnosia for stimuli with nameable and unnameable parts, associating the former with alexia and the latter with prosopagnosia. Corballis (in press) proposes that the left hemisphere is specialized for part-based representations in language, imagery, and object recognition, which he conjectures are evolutionarily recent representations. Therefore, in his framework the present distinction could be phrased in terms of evolutionarily newer versus older recognition mechanisms. In addition to left versus right hemisphere, nameable versus nonnameable and evolutionarily recent versus old, there are undoubtedly other ways that one could cast the distinction between agnosia without alexia and agnosia without prosopagnosia. Whatever interpretation ultimately seems most appropriate, the data currently available suggest that the range of associative agnosias can be accounted for by postulating just two underlying visual abilities. Furthermore, the pattern of neuropathology in these cases seems to respect the two-category structure being proposed here.

5.6 Optic Aphasia

Given the conclusion reached earlier in this chapter, that associative agnosia and optic aphasia are distinct phenomena, the question now arises of how to interpret optic aphasia. What sorts of representations and processes underlie our normal ability to name visual stimuli, and which of these has been damaged in optic aphasia? At first glance the answer seems perfectly obvious: Optic aphasia appears to be a cut-and-dried case of a disconnection syndrome, in which intact vision centers are separated from intact naming centers. However, on closer examination of the abilities and deficits of these patients, optic aphasia poses a serious paradox, which is difficult to dispell within the framework of conventional models of visual naming.

It is generally assumed that the functional architecture underlying visual naming must include three major components: vision, semantics, and language. Exactly what these three terms mean in this context may not be entirely clear, but the gist of such an account must surely be correct in the following sense. In order to name a visually presented object, I must see it clearly enough to be able to access some semantic information about it (i.e., to know what it is), and once I know what it is I must then retrieve and produce its name. Surprisingly, there is no part of this model that can be damaged to produce optic aphasia. Given that optic aphasics can gesture appropriately to visual stimuli they cannot name, and correctly sort or match visual stimuli according to semantic attributes, then their impairment cannot lie anywhere in vision, semantics, or the path between the two. Given that they can supply the appropriate name to verbal definitions, sounds, and palpated objects, then their impairment cannot lie anywhere in semantics, naming operations, or the path between the two. Note that all possible loci for damage in this simple model of visual naming have just been eliminated!

5.6.1 A direct route for object naming

In order to account for optic aphasia, various alterations have been proposed for the model just outlined. Ratcliff and Newcombe (1982) surveyed the problem and suggested that the least unappealing solution is to postulate a direct route from vision to naming. According to this model, shown in figure 27, in addition to semantically mediated object naming, there is also a nonsemantic route whereby specific visual percepts can evoke their corresponding name directly. In normal visual naming, the two routes are used in parallel and together produce accurate, reliable naming. In optic aphasia, the direct route has been interrupted, and the loss of this redundancy decreases the reliability of the system. While acknowledging that the solution is somewhat ad hoc, these authors also point out that a similar direct route has been postulated for reading, to account for deep dyslexia, and that in this case independent evidence for it exists: Schwartz, Saffran, and Marin (1980) described a patient who was able to read aloud, including irregular words such as "leopard," without appearing to know what they meant. This is consistent with the loss of the semantic route for reading and the preservation of the nonsemantic route. As Ratcliff and Newcombe point out, however, the analogous case for visual object naming—a patient who can name visually presented objects without knowing what they are—has never been described. Furthermore, chronometric research in

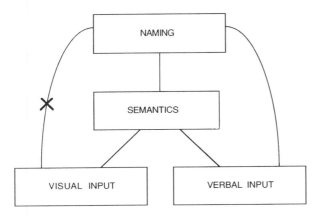

Figure 27
A cognitive architecture for explaining optic aphasia, with a direct route from vision to naming, based on the ideas of Ratcliff and Newcombe (1982).

cognitive psychology has demonstrated that even after extensive practice, picture naming invariably requires an additional processing stage, mediating between visual perception and naming, which is not required for word naming (i.e., reading aloud; e.g., Theios and Amrhein, 1989).

5.6.2 Modality-specific semantic systems

Another way to account for optic aphasia is to postulate multiple semantic systems, each associated with a different modality. Beauvois (1982) proposed that optic aphasia can be explained as a disconnection between visual and verbal semantics, as shown in figure 28. Although she did not define these two terms explicitly, her discussion of them implies that visual semantics consists of imagerylike visual information about objects, which can be accessed by stimuli of any modality, and verbal semantics consists of verbal associations and abstract properties of objects that cannot be visualized or represented concretely in any particular modality, also accessible by stimuli of any modality. This subdivision of semantics by modality works well to explain the phenomena described by Beauvois and Saillant (1985) in a case of "optic aphasia for colors." The patient, M.P., was unable to name colors or to perform a variety of other tasks in which color names must be associated with color percepts. In contrast, M.P. was able to perform color tasks that required either verbal-verbal or visual-visual associations. For example, she was unable to recall the color of an object on spoken request (e.g., "What color is a gherkin?"), because the verbally posed question had to be interpreted using verbal semantics, whereas the answer had to be retrieved from

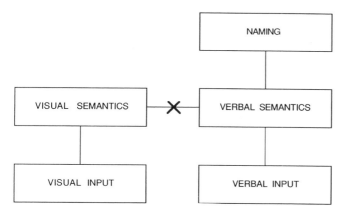

Figure 28
A cognitive architecture for explaining optic aphasia with separate modality-specific semantic systems, based on the ideas of Beauvois (1982).

visual semantics. In contrast, she was able to retrieve color names when they were merely verbal associates of a concept, as opposed to part of the visual semantics of a concept (e.g., "What color name would you give to communists?"). In addition, she was able to report the colors of objects when the question was posed nonverbally, by having her point to the correctly colored version in a set of pictures of an object. Note that this task requires the same kind of information to be retrieved as the first task mentioned, but in contrast to the first task, verbal semantics are not needed to understand the question. Although Beauvois's idea of modality-specific semantic systems does an excellent job of accounting for the patterns of performance in patient M.P. with color tasks, it does not account well for the broader range of phenomena that consititute the syndrome of optic aphasia. For example, the ability of optic aphasics to sort visually dissimilar objects into superordinate categories and to match visually presented objects based on function (e.g., a button and a zipper) cannot be explained by a disconnection between visual and verbal semantics, unless the term "visual semantics" is expanded to mean more than just knowledge of the visual appearances of objects, to include all the knowledge that one has about an object, including the functions it serves, the sounds it makes, its categorical relations with superordinate concepts, and so on, short of its name per se. On this reading of the term "visual semantics," what makes it visual is that it is accessed only by visually presented stimuli. The notion that we have multiple "copies" of our entire stock of semantic knowledge, one for each modality of stimulus presentation, seems quite ad hoc, not to mention unparsimonious.

5.6.3 Optic Aphasia as 'semantic access agnosia'

Riddoch and Humphreys (1987b) suggest an interpretation of optic aphasia according to which semantics is a unitary entity. They place the processing deficit between vision and semantics, as shown in figure 29. Accordingly, they classify optic aphasia as a kind of agnosia, which they call 'semantic access agnosia', because vision is normal but there is difficulty accessing semantic information with the products of visual perception. This conception of optic aphasia coincides with the traditional conception of associative agnosia, as "normal perception, stripped of its meaning." The question is, how well does this conception of optic aphasia account for the abilities and deficits of optic aphasics? On the face of things, Riddoch and Humphreys's account seems to predict rather different behavior than has in fact been observed in optic aphasia, these differences amounting to just the differences between associative agnosia and optic aphasia outlined in the previous chapter. Optic aphasics can categorize visually dissimilar stimuli according to their superordinate and functional relatedness, and produce appropriate gestures in response to a visual stimulus. How is this possible if access from vision to semantics is impaired? Riddoch and Humphreys address the problems of categorizing and gesturing separately.

Riddoch and Humphreys's account of optic aphasia predicts poor performance on semantic categorization tasks with visually presented stimuli, and yet optic aphasics have generally been found to do well on these tasks. In defense of their account, Riddoch and Humphreys point out that these categorization tasks have typically been quite easy, such

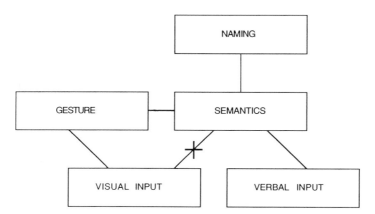

Figure 29
A cognitive architecture for explaining optic aphasia as a disconnection between vision and semantics, based on the ideas of Riddoch and Humphreys (1986).

that some residual ability to access semantics might be sufficient to perform the categorizations but insufficient for precise naming. Consistent with this hypothesis, their patient did well on a task of grouping objects into superordinate categories, but performed poorly on a different categorization task, which they suggested tests semantic access more stringently. In two other cases of optic aphasia there has been the suggestion of impaired semantic processing of visually presented stimuli on difficult tasks: Lhermitte and Beauvois noted that when Jules F. was asked to point to a named picture that was not present in the array of pictures, he would point to a semantically related picture rather than say the item was missing. The patient of Gil et al. (1985) performed poorly on a task that involved matching pictures according to "metaphorical" relatedness. These findings are consistent with Riddoch and Humphreys's hypothesis that semantic access is impaired, although another possible interpretation should be noted as well: In the two instances of more stringent categorization tasks, the associations between items are encoded in language, and are not available from nonverbal forms of knowledge. This is true of the Gil et al. metaphorical relations task, and is true of at least a portion of Riddoch and Humphreys's materials, which relied on verbal associates such as cup and saucer, apples and oranges, or on name similarity to break "ties" between alternative plausible pairings, such as candle and light bulb versus candle and candle holder (the correct pairing). Thus, it is possible that specifically verbal knowledge must be consulted in order to do well on these tasks. The finding that Jules F. selected semantic associates of the designated target when the target was absent is difficult to interpret, as he may not have realized that saying "it isn't here" was an option.

A second apparent difficulty for the semantic access account of optic aphasia is that optic aphasics can produce appropriate gestures to visually presented objects that they cannot name, suggesting that they have accessed semantics. Riddoch and Humphreys argue that gesturing is a misleading measure of semantic access for two reasons: First, gestures are inherently less precise than names and are therefore a less precise means of testing comprehension. To use an example provided by Ratcliff and Newcombe (1982), the gestures for a sock and a shoe are virtually identical, whereas the names are highly discriminable and a patient who said "sock" when shown a shoe would be considered to have made a semantic error. Although this is true, it cannot alone account for the difference in gesturing and naming performance in optic aphasia. For example, Lhermitte and Beauvois (1973) report that their patient made no gesturing errors at all for a large set of stimuli, which were misnamed over a quarter of the time. Furthermore, this discrepancy does not seem attributable to the greater ambiguity of gesture, as the incorrect names do not generally correspond to a similar gesture (e.g., in response to a boot, a correct gesture to indicate a boot and the word "hat").

A second reason Riddoch and Humphreys give for discounting correct gestures as evidence for semantic access is that an object's physical appearance alone is often sufficient to dictate what the appropriate gesture might be. This idea is similar to what Gibson (1979) termed "affordances," in the sense that a certain shape will afford grasping with certain hand shapes and not others, will afford motion in certain directions more easily than in others, and so on. Although it is true that the physical appearance of an object can certainly reduce the number of possible gestures that a subject must consider, for example the shape of an orange is incompatible with hand-shapes for holding thin objects such as cigarettes, it seems wrong to conclude that the appearance of an object constrains the possible gestures to the degree that gesturing ability could be intact when objects are not recognized (i.e., when their semantics are not accessed). After all, there are many examples of similar-looking objects that have very different gestures associated with them: a needle and a tooth pick, an eraser and a piece of taffy, a chopstick and a swizzlestick, etc.

5.6.4 Superadditive impairments in vision and naming

The paradox of optic aphasia arises because we cannot identify a single locus, within the simple three-part architecture of vision, semantics, and naming, that could be damaged to account for the abilities and impairments of optic aphasics. One possible resolution to this paradox is that more than one locus must be damaged in order to produce optic aphasia. Figure 30 shows two loci where partial damage would impair the naming of visual stimuli more than the nonverbal identification of visual stimuli through gesture or the naming of nonvisual stimuli such as verbally described objects, because twice as much damage contributes to performance of the former than the latter tasks. So far, this account falls short of explaining optic aphasia because it does not address the *disproportionality* of the visual naming deficit relative to vision and naming as assessed in other ways in these patients. The probability of success in visual naming is not simply the product of the probabilities of success in nonverbal tests of vision and nonvisual tests of naming. Vision and naming per se seem near-normal in these patients, and yet visual naming is grossly impaired. Therefore, in order to explain optic aphasia by damage at two separate loci, one must assume that effects of the damage are superadditive.

Is it completely ad hoc to suppose that the effects of damage at two separate loci would be superadditive? There are, in fact, two types of consideration that provide independent support for this assumption.

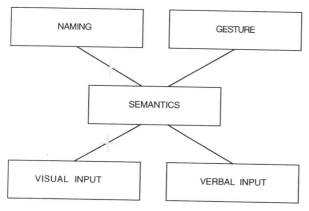

Figure 30
A cognitive architecture for explaining optic aphasia with superadditive effects of damage at two loci.

The first is a computational consideration. The massively parallel constraint satisfaction architectures described in section 5.1.3 have the ability to complete or recover partially damaged or degraded input representations, provided the damage is not too great. For example, in the McClelland and Rumelhart word perception model described in section 3.3.1, the same mechanisms that give rise to the "word superiority effect" will help restore a missing or degraded letter: The interactions among the representations of that letter, the surrounding letters, and stored words will result in the eventual activation of that letter representation as fully as if it had been presented intact. However, if too many letters are degraded, or if a letter is too severely degraded, there will come a point where the system cannot restore the information that is lacking.

It is conceivable that when a task involves activating just one damaged part of the system, the noisy output of that part can be restored, or "cleaned up," by the remaining intact network, but that when two damaged parts of the system must operate together, with the noisy output from one damaged subsystem being the input to another damaged subsystem, the recovery capabilities of the network will be exceeded, and performance will drop precipitously. This is plausible given the extreme nonlinear behavior of massively parallel constraint satisfaction networks (Lapedes and Farber, 1987). Of course, it must be tested empirically by building and damaging such a system, a project currently underway.[3]

A second reason for suspecting that damage to two separate loci might have superadditive effects comes from an intriguing study by Bisiach (1966). He asked a group of anomic patients to name pictures of common objects, and if they could not name them, to convey their recognition of them in some other way, such as gesturing or circumlocuting. The pictures were either full-color paintings, line drawings, or line drawings with stray marks superimposed. Although the subjects were not agnosic, their naming performance was poorest for the marked up drawings, next poorest for the normal drawings, and best for the full-color paintings. Their recognition performance, while also somewhat influenced by the visual quality of the stimulus, did not account for all of the difference in naming performance. That is, the naming ability per se of patients with anomia is influenced by the nature of the visual input. One way of looking at Bisiach's experiment is that he induced optic aphasia by taking patients with damage to the naming system, and simulating the effect of damage to a second locus, visual processing, by giving them low-quality stimuli.

5.6.5 Hemisphere-specific semantic systems

The foregoing accounts of optic aphasia all share the characteristic that they draw exclusively on the explanatory "machinery" of cognitive psychology: They are all cast in terms of the same representations and processes that have been postulated by cognitive psychologists studying intact brains using response time methods and the like. In particular, the two different architectures for "semantics" invoked in these explanations of optic aphasia come from the two main schools of thought on modality-specificity of knowledge representation in cognitive psychology: The idea of a unified form of semantic memory that figures in the direct route, semantic access, and superadditive impairment hypotheses has its roots in the work of cognitive psychologists such as Anderson (1976) and Pylyshyn (1984), and the idea of distinct visual and verbal semantic memory modules, found in the multiple semantic systems hypothesis, has its roots in the work of cognitive psychologists such as Allport (1980) and Paivio (1971).

A very different account of optic aphasia, shown in figure 31, was recently proposed by Coslett and Saffran (1989), and includes a third kind of architecture for semantics. In this model, semantics is subdivided by *hemisphere*, a distinction that has no direct analog in cognitive psychology. They suggest that optic aphasia is a disconnection syndrome whereby the products of normal visual processing cannot access the left hemisphere's semantic system, but can access the right hemisphere's semantic system. This account is explanatory to the extent that we have some independent information about the semantic systems of the two hemispheres, which match the abilities and deficits of optic aphasics. In fact, the correspondence is striking. Right hemisphere semantics appear

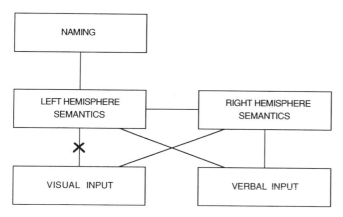

Figure 31
A cognitive architecture for explaining optic aphasia with separate hemisphere-specific semantic systems, based on the ideas of Coslett and Saffran (1989).

to be less finely differentiated than left hemisphere semantics (Zaidel, 1985), accounting for semantic errors in naming, as well as the combination of good performance on categorization tasks that test broad superordinate categories and poor performance on the more stringent tests of categorization. In addition, Coslett and Saffran present a detailed analysis of their patient's residual reading abilities, which closely matches the known profile of right hemisphere reading abilities: He was able to match auditorily presented nouns but not functors or nonwords to printed words, and was insensitive to affixes. There is thus independent reason to believe that in this case, at least, visual input was being interpreted by the right hemisphere.

Chapter 6
Conclusions

A remarkable variety of visual disorders can arise from damage confined to the cortical visual areas at the back of the brain. The sheer diversity of these disorders suggests a complex organization for higher vision and presents us with an opportunity for some cognitive neuropsychological bootstrapping: To infer properties of the organization of normal vision from the array of visual disorders that follow brain damage, and at the same time to identify the underlying impairment in the disorders, in terms of components of the normal system that have been damaged. This is what I have tried to do in the preceding chapters. In this final chapter, I will present a distillation of some of the more general implications of my conclusions for neuropsychology and cognitive science.

6.1 Neuropsychological Taxonomies

Recent discussions of method in cognitive neuropsychology have warned against the danger of grouping patients for study (e.g., Caramazza, 1984). In fact, the arguments given against grouping patients are actually arguments against grouping them incorrectly. Traditional neuropsychological group study designs, in which patients are grouped on the basis of hemisphere or quadrant of brain damage or performance on psychometric or clinical tests, are not appropriate for answering most questions about cognitive processes: These groups will be heterogeneous with respect to the impairments that are the subject of study, and we therefore risk basing our conclusions on average performance profiles that are artifactual, in that they may not exist in any one case. Of course, the fact that inappropriate categorization of patients can lead one astray is not an argument against categorization per se. Theories are statements about categories of things. Even if the theory is proposed on the basis of observing one unique thing, it is not about a unique thing. Therefore, theories and taxonomies go hand in hand, and it will be impossible to have a correct theory unless one also has a correct system of categories.

In the neuropsychology of visual object recognition, I have argued that many researchers have grouped patients incorrectly. In some cases, impairments that are different in kind are grouped together as different manifestations or degrees of the same underlying impairment. For example, patients with two very distinct disorders have been called simultanagnosics and discussed interchangeably by many authors. These patients have also been lumped with yet a third group of patients, apperceptive agnosics, by some authors. Prosopagnosics have been assumed by many to have a milder form of the across-the-board agnosia in which patients cannot read. Optic aphasics and associative agnosics have been grouped together, sometimes with the optic aphasia treated as a mild form of associative agnosia. In the preceding chapters, I have shown why, on purely empirical, "bottom-up" grounds, these patients should be put in separate categories for purposes of theory development. In other cases, standard categories include distinctions between disorders that may well be different manifestations or degrees of the same underlying impairment. For example, I have argued that pure alexia and ventral simultanagnosia may represent the same impairment, again, on purely empirical grounds. These taxonomic decisions are prerequisite for making the theoretical inferences also proposed in the preceding chapters, from discerning the role of objects and locations in the allocation of visual attention to considering whether noninnate skills might be carried out using dedicated neural hardware.

I have stressed the importance of delineating categories of patients using purely empirical criteria, both behavioral and neuroanatomical, and have segregated my discussions of the *categories* of impairment and my discussion of the theoretical *interpretations* of these categories into different chapters in order to emphasize this point. Of course, it is probably impossible to launder all implicit theory out of our observations. The suggestion is simply to try as best we can to minimize its role in structuring an initial taxonomy. Doesn't this run counter to the goals of the new field of cognitive neuropsychology, to put more cognitive theory into neuropsychology and to leave behind the atheoretical, descriptive approaches of the past? If we had a theory of visual object recognition that we knew to be correct, then it would of course be worth using that theory in sorting out individual cases into categories, to discriminate the relevant similarities and differences from the irrelevant ones. However, one of the primary reasons for studying disorders of object recognition is that we do not yet have a theory of how it works, and we hope to derive some ideas and constraints for such a theory from these disorders. In such a context, basing one's taxonomy on a *wrong* theory is much worse than on no theory at all. This is particularly true when we use a theory to structure the data base that we then turn around and use as evidence for the theory, and it is even more particularly true when the data base is as "messy" as the case material of neuropsychology: All cases of brain damage have many aspects that are irrelevant to whatever scientific question is being asked, and it is therefore permissible (in fact, practically necessary) to ignore much of the information available about any particular case. Neuropsychological data are also "messy" in that patients' abilities after brain damage are not all-or-none, and a judgement call is often required to decide whether a certain level of performance should be viewed as impaired or not. In grouping patients into categories according to what we take to be the important and relevant similarities and differences, we implicitly decide which aspects of the cases can be ignored and which abilities should be considered impaired. As these are decisions that may well vary according to one's theory, then the introduction of theory at the stage of taxonomizing will act as a filter, de-emphasizing or even eliminating aspects of the data that could be useful in testing that theory or other theories.

For example, Bay's (1953) theory of object recognition, discussed in chapter 1, included only two types of processes, elementary visual perception and amodal general intellectual abilities, and he invariably found that patients with object recognition difficulties could be grouped into one or both of two categories: those with impaired elementary visual perception and those with impaired general intellectual ability. Lissauer (1890/1988) formulated the apperceptive/associative agnosia distinction primarily on the basis of an a priori theory of object recognition, rather than on the basis of clinical observation. The categorization of agnosia that follows from this theoretical framework has remained in use for over a hundred years, during which time many cases have been categorized as having associative agnosia, or in Teuber's words, "normal perception stripped of its meaning." However, in chapters 4 and 5 we saw that the available data on the perceptual capabilities of associative agnosics, including object agnosics, prosopagnosics, and pure alexics, fails to support the idea that perception is normal in these cases. On the contrary, perception appears to be impaired in characteristic ways in these patients. It seems likely that the lack of attention paid to the visual impairments of associative agnosics results from the theoretical idea, implicit in the traditional taxonomy of agnosia, that visual abnormalities are not the cause of their recognition impairment. As a result, the implications of these patients' perceptual difficulties for the nature of object recognition (e.g., the computational architectures discussed in sections 5.1.2 and 5.1.3) have not been considered. There has also been little research effort aimed at characterizing these visual impairments and hence inferring the nature of high-level visual representations underlying object recognition. In short, theoretical progress has been inhibited by bringing the wrong theories into the research too early, at the stage of taxonomizing.

Probably the most sophisticated attempt to impose a theory-based taxonomy on disorders of visual object recognition was made by Humphreys and Riddoch (1987b). They motivate their taxonomy by stating that "To draw any implications from . . . patients for normal vision, their deficits need to be classified according to the process(es) which are disrupted" (p. 282), and suggest a taxonomy "based partly on reported behavioral differences between patients, and also partly on a theoretical framework [shown in figure 23]" (p. 299). But inevitably, at this stage of theoretical progress, there is some degree of strain between the groupings dictated by behavioral data and those dictated by the theoretical framework, and the latter tend to predominate. For example, damage to part (d) of their framework corresponds to loss of the stored knowledge about the form of objects, with intact perceptual representations (and semantic knowledge), a combination of abilities and impairments that has yet to be demonstrated. Conversely, for example, there is no place in the taxonomy for a distinction that does seem empirically real, the dissociation between disorders of face recognition and disorders of printed word recognition. As a result, users of this taxonomy are unlikely even to consider certain important theoretical issues such as the computational architecture underlying object recognition, already mentioned in connection with Lissauer's taxonomy, or the unity versus the modularity of object representations (e.g., for faces, words, common objects).

6.2 The Functional Architecture and Neuroanatomic Correlates of Visual Object Recognition: A Preliminary Sketch Based on the Available Neuropsychological Evidence

6.2.1 The grouped array
Higher vision, as revealed by the agnosias, begins with the grouping of local elements of the visual field into larger-scale contours, regions, and/ or surfaces. Apperceptive agnosics show us what vision is like without these grouping processes. Their perception of local contour, color, and brightness is relatively preserved, and yet they have a severe impairment in the perception of overall form. What is meant by "overall form" includes even the simplest geometric properties that require combining information across local regions of the visual field. For example, the ability to see that the two halves of a line with a small break between them belong to the same form is impaired in these patients. Perhaps not surprisingly, these patients have difficulty in matching shapes, recognizing them, and selectively attending to them. The implication of this

constellation of abilities and impairments for the functional architecture of object recognition seems straightforward: There is a stage (or stages) of vision in which the separately registered local elements of the visual field are grouped into higher-order geometric representations, and that this stage is prerequisite for virtually all higher visual processing. The one exception may concern the perception of nonlocal geometry through motion. The fact that some of these patients benefit rather dramatically from stimulus movement implies that the grouping of local elements may occur by the correlated nature of their motion independently of grouping based on static features of the visual field. As discussed in chapter 2, the damage to these patients' brains is generally fairly diffuse, although occipital damage is common to all and seems most likely to be the critical component in producing this syndrome. Therefore, grouping is presumably a function of the occipital lobes.

There is no evidence that the grouping processes can be modulated by top-down influences, either by familiarity of the stimulus configuration or directed attention. With other types of patients, for example dorsal and ventral simultanagnosics, we have seen evidence that the underlying impairment is in processes that can be modulated by knowledge and by selective attention: Whether a dorsal simultanagnosic sees just one dot or one rectangle made up of many dots is partly under the patient's conscious control. How many objects a ventral simultanagnosic can recognize in a brief presentation depends upon their familiarity, and which objects the patient recognizes depends upon the conscious deployment of spatial selective attention. In contrast, there are no reports of apperceptive agnosics perceiving familiar shapes better than unfamiliar ones, or perceiving shapes better when they know which shape to look for or where to look for it. For example, the patient of Landis et al. (1982) perceived the stimulus shown in figure 4 as the number *7415*, a number with no particular significance, rather than the highly familiar visual pattern *THIS*. The factors that determine an apperceptive agnosic's perception seem exclusively tied to the physical properties of the stimuli: whether there are breaks in the lines or superimposed marks, whether the lines are curved or straight, whether the stimulus is moving, and so on. Of course, lack of evidence is not grounds for firm conclusions, especially when the data base is so sketchy and anecdotal. Therefore, we can draw only a tentative conclusion regarding the directions of information flow at this stage of vision. That tentative conclusion is that the process whereby the local, separately registered elements of the visual field are grouped into larger contours, regions, and/or surfaces is a purely stimulus-driven process. It takes a very circumscribed range of input, which presumably includes the local spatial relations among these visual elements, and which excludes considerations of whether a particular grouping would yield a recognizable figure or whether a particular grouping falls within an attended region of space. This tentative hypothesis is represented in figure 32 by having the arrows between the array of local visual elements and the grouped array pointing in one direction only.

6.2.2 Interactions between the grouped array, spatial attention and object representations

The array of grouped stimulus elements interacts with two higher-level systems: the spatial attention system and the object recognition system. Dorsal simultanagnosia represents a disruption of the spatial system, in which the contents of the grouped array that can be attended to in a given amount of time is abnormally limited. Ventral simultanagnosia represents a disruption of the object recognition system, in which the contents of the grouped array that can be recognized in a given amount of time is abnormally limited. The critical lesion sites for these disorders imply that the parietal and/or anterior superior occipital cortex is involved in spatial attention, and the left inferior temporo-occipital cortex plays a special role in object recognition.

Certain characteristics of dorsal and ventral simultanagnosia seem to have paradoxical implications concerning the relations between the spatial attention and object recognition systems. On the one hand, there is strong neuropsychological evidence that the spatial attention and object recognition systems operate independently and in parallel, as impairments in each of these systems is dissociable from impairments in the other. Dorsal simultanagnosics have normal object recognition capability; so long as they can see an object, they can recognize it. This is true even of multipart objects such as words, which are difficult for ventral simultanagnosics. Ventral simultanagnosics have normal spatial attention, whereas their object recognition is slowed; they can see and orient to stimuli occurring anywhere in the visual field. If these systems were arranged in series, that is, if either of them provided necessary input to the other, then these disorders would not be doubly dissociable.

On the other hand, there is evidence that appears to suggest that the two systems are arranged in series. The fact that the attentional limitation in dorsal simultanagnosics is at least partly a function of number of *objects* (determined by familiarity and not merely low-level physical stimulus properties) would seem to imply that the spatial attention system is operating on input that has already been processed by the object recognition system. In addition, there is evidence that seems to imply the opposite serial organization! The fact that ventral simultanagnosics benefit from spatial cuing would seem to imply that input to the object recognition system is gated by spatial attention.

This apparent paradox can be explained by the architecture shown in figure 32, in which spatial attention and object recognition do indeed operate in parallel on the grouped array. The interactions between each of the higher-level systems and the grouped array are described below. Although the account is frankly underspecified and perhaps also under-determined by the available data, it has the virtue of accounting for the effects of object representations on spatial attention and the effects of spatial attention on object recognition with the simple arrangement shown in figure 32, without invoking any assumptions not already motivated by a consideration of the separate functions of the spatial attention and object recognition systems.

The spatial attention system can select portions of the grouped array, either by top-down means (i.e., the person decides to selectively attend to a portion of the grouped array) or because of activity in the grouped array (e.g., the onset or movement of a stimulus). What does it mean for a portion of the grouped array to be "selected"? Consistent with the standard usage of this term in theories of selective attention (e.g., Posner, Snyder, and Davidson, 1980; Triesman and Gelade, 1980), stimuli occurring in this region will be more likely to be detected, and they will be more likely to be recognized by the object recognition system (which, because it is hypothesized to have limited capacity, cannot recognize all objects at once). Selection is presumably accomplished by adding activation to the attended region of the grouped array.[1]

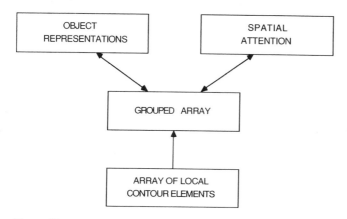

Figure 32
A sketch of the relations among two kinds of array representations of the visual field, spatial attention and object representations, inferred from the neuropsychological data.

The object recognition system redescribes portions of the grouped array in a more abstract format, which captures the invariant three-dimensional geometric properties of the distal stimulus object more fully than the array-format representation. In terms of its interactions with the grouped array, this requires that the object recognition system divide the surfaces, regions, and/or contours of the grouped array into portions that correspond to the image of a single object. The task of parsing the array in terms of one's knowledge of possible objects involves a potential chicken-and-egg problem, in that a bit of contour may or may not constitute the boundary of an object, depending upon the candidate objects, while an object may or may not be a candidate, depending upon the boundaries visible in the array. As discussed in section 5.1.3, problems such as this in which multiple constraints must be satisfied simultaneously are well suited to connectionist computational architectures. In the present case, an obvious solution would be analogous to McClelland and Rumelhart's word-recognition model, discussed in section 3.3.1, in which lower-level representations (in this case groupings in the array) activate candidate higher-level representations (in this case object representations), and the activated higher-level representations simultaneously activate their corresponding lower-level representations. If this were the case, then collections of surfaces, regions, and/or contours in the grouped array that correspond to objects will receive top-down support from the object recognition system.

The effects of spatial attention on the object recognition ability of ventral simultanagnosics, and the effect of object representations on the allocation of attention in dorsal simultanagnosics, can now be explained. According to the picture just sketched, there are three sources of activation in the grouped array, determining which portions of it will be active: bottom-up activation from stimuli, top-down activation from the spatial attention system, and top-down activation from the object recognition system of regions corresponding to parsed objects. The ability of ventral simultanagnosics to recognize a stimulus at a spatially cued location, among many other stimuli at different locations, can be explained by supposing that the cue leads patients to allocate spatial attention to the region of the grouped array containing the object to be recognized. The additional activation causes the object at that location to be encoded first by the object recognition system. Because ventral simultanagnosics are hypothesized to have sufficient object recognition capacity to recognize a single object, the spatially cued object will be recognized.

Similarly, it is possible to explain the role of objects in the attentional limitation of dorsal simultanagnosics by the effect of object representations on the activity in the grouped array. In the course of interactive parsing of the grouped array, the object recognition system will tend to activate regions of the array that correspond to objects. As the spatial attention system will be engaged by activity in the grouped array, this will result in attention being engaged by regions of the array that correspond to objects. Assuming that the underlying impairment in dorsal simultanagnosia is one of disengaging attention, as discussed in section 3.2.1, the attention will stay stuck to one region of the grouped array, which will generally correspond to a whole object because of the top-down activation from their intact object recognition systems. The occasional object recognition difficulties of these patients occur when a portion of an object captures their attention. In the framework outlined here, this corresponds to an incorrect parse of the grouped array being maintained by their "sticky" attention. Note that this account of the role of objects in visual attention is quite different from previous object-based attentional theories, in which attention is said to be object-based *as opposed to location-based*, and to operate relatively late in visual processing, on representations of objects per se (e.g., Duncan, 1984). In the current framework, attention operates on relatively low-level, array-format representations, and is fundamentally location-based. Nevertheless, it accounts for the findings that have typically been taken to support object-based attention theories (section 3.2.2).

6.2.3 Object recognition

Neuropsychological data can also shed light on the internal workings of the object recognition system. There are two main issues that can be addressed using the available evidence from agnosia. The first is the issue of modularity within the domain of visual object representation. Are all objects recognized the same way, or are there specialized subsystems? If there are subsystems, how are they individuated, and what is the division of labor between them? The second concerns the implementation of object recognition in the brain. Are object representations local or distributed, and what kind of computational architecture underlies the process of recognition?

The dissociations among face recognition, printed word recognition, and object recognition suggest that there are different types of object recognition processes, which may be required to greater and lesser extents by these different classes of objects. The analysis of the patterns of cooccurrence presented in section 5.5 suggests that there may be just two underlying types of recognition ability damaged in associative agnosia, one required primarily for written words and to a lesser extent for other objects, and one required primarily for faces and to a lesser extent for other objects. A tentative interpretation for these two underlying forms of object recognition is as follows: One involves the capacity to represent multiple shapes, required for word recognition as well as for the recognition of other objects that undergo decomposition into multiple parts (and whose identity cannot be inferred after just one or two parts have been encoded). This ability depends upon the left inferior temporo-occipital region. The other involves the capacity to represent the parts themselves, which will be particularly taxed when an object does not undergo much decomposition in the course of object recognition and therefore has fairly complex parts. It was argued that faces are the prime example of this type of object, although certain other objects such as animals and makes of automobile probably also share this property. The representation of the parts themselves appears to depend upon temporo-occipital cortex bilaterally.

Whatever the basis for the different object recognition abilities that we see dissociated in prosopagnosia, pure alexia, and object agnosia, it seems likely to be a function of the visual properties of stimuli, and not their semantic category. Although prosopagnosics are often said to have difficulty recognizing "living things," and pure alexics' impairment is mainly evident with "verbal material," more careful testing has revealed that the impairments do not respect the boundaries of these semantic categories: For example, prosopagnosics also have difficulty recognizing buildings and automobiles, and pure alexics show slowed recognition of multiple shapes from any semantic category. Reports of bona fide semantic impairments were found to involve post-perceptual processing, insofar as these impairments affect performance in purely verbal and memory tasks as well as visual recognition tasks. As argued in section 5.4.1, this implies that semantic knowledge is not used in deriving a representation of an object's shape for purposes of recognition.

The implementation of visual object recognition in the brain seems most consistent with a parallel distributed processing architecture, both in the nature of its representations and the way in which those representations are searched during recognition. Whereas naming impairments can be confined to categories as specific as fruits and vegetables, implying that these representations are implemented relatively locally in neural hardware (section 5.4.2), visual recognition impairments are fairly broad, implying that the underlying representations are distributed. A particular face might be represented by a pattern of activity distributed over a large number of neurons, many of which might also be active during the representation of a different face, and possibly even objects other than faces. The way in which stimuli are matched against stored knowledge of object appearances also seems consistent with parallel distributed computation. As discussed in sections 5.1.2 and 5.1.3,

Notes

Chapter 3

1. They have also been taken to imply that there are no capacity limitations in character recognition. However, it is more accurate to say that, if they exist, capacity limitations are not reached with the small numbers of characters used in this research.
2. The hypothesis that there are two kinds of recognition ability, one of which is taxed more by faces than by words, and the other of which is taxed more by words than by faces, will be considered in section 5.5.

Chapter 4

1. A number of patients who appear to be associative visual agnosics by all other criteria are impaired at tactile object recognition (e.g., Feinberg, Rothi and Heilman, 1986; Ratcliff and Newcombe, 1982; Taylor and Warrington, 1971). This association may result from incidental damage to tactile association areas, or it may reflect the use of visual mediation in tactile object recognition by some patients.
2. Nielsen (1937) reviewed a large set of cases with visual agnosia following unilateral brain damage, drawn primarily from the German neurological literature of the decades just before and after the turn of the century. He concluded that a unilateral lesion in the visual areas of the dominant (usually left) hemisphere was sufficient to cause agnosia. This conclusion must be tempered by two additional considerations: First, Nielsen sampled only unilateral cases. The fact that most cases of associative agnosia have bilateral damage to the visual areas suggests that the minor hemisphere damage in these cases cannot be viewed as an irrelevant lesion coincidentally superimposed on the critically lesioned brain. Second, many of the cases reviewed by Nielsen had severe language and perceptual problems, raising the possibility that all were not "pure" cases of associative agnosia.
3. M.D. did show a mild impairment on a sorting task in which 75 pictures of fruits, vegetables, other food products, animals, and vehicles were to be placed in piles according to their different categories. His error rate was certainly lower in this task than in the naming tasks (about 20 percent compared to about 40 percent for simple naming), but still poses somewhat of a mystery given the ostensibly nonverbal nature of the task. It is conceivable that categorization is aided by covert verbal labelling. This is consistent with the observations that aphasic patients do poorly on category sorting tasks, and paradoxically worse with pictures than with words, despite no signs of agnosic behavior in everyday life (McCleary and Hirst, 1986).

Chapter 5

1. They go on to consider the possibility that simultaneous form perception per se is at fault, and present data they take to imply intact simultaneous form perception.   Unfortunately, the task that they use to test simultaneous form perception is unlike any of the others used previously in the literature, and appears not to require simultaneous form perception: A string of letters (length 4-8) is presented, which is either composed of all the same letter or has one odd letter out, and the subjects' task is to discriminate the homogeneous letter strings from the letter strings with a single odd letter. Such a task can be performed without identifying each component letter, but by merely detecting nonuniformities in the distribution of visual features.   In effect, the task is a texture boundary detection task, which for most pairs of letters can be performed preattentively (Triesman and Gelade, 1980).

2. Some cases published as cases of associative agnosia seem, in fact, to be cases of optic aphasia according to the criteria discussed in section 4.5, and are therefore not included in table 1.   These cases are: Ferro and Santos (1984); Hecaen, Goldblum, Masure, and Ramier (1974); Morin, Rivrain, Eustache, Lambert, and Courtheoux (1984); Mouren, Tatossian, Trupheme, Guidicelli, and Fresco (1967), and Rouzaud, Dumas, Degiovanni, Larmande, Ployet, and Laffont (1978). However, even if these cases were included they would not change the conclusions to be reported.

3. With the collaboration of Mike Lewicki, Paddy McMullen, and David Plaut.

Chapter 6

1. This is consistent with the effects of attention on the sensitivity and threshold of normal subjects in tasks requiring detection and identification of visual stimuli.   Adding activation to a region of the grouped array would merely change the effective threshold for detection of stimuli occurring in that region, as less bottom-up activation coming into the array from the stimulus would be needed to reach a given threshold of activation in the array. However, on the assumption that the limited-capacity object recognition system operates preferentially on the most active regions of the array, then the addition of activation to a region of the grouped array would result in preferential processing of stimuli in that region by the object recognition system, leading (not implausibly, at least) to increased discriminability or sensitivity for identification of those stimuli. Shaw (1984) and Muller and Findlay (1987) found just this pattern in their research with normal subjects: Selective spatial attention affects only the threshold for detection of stimuli, but affects the discriminability of stimuli in tasks requiring identification.

Glossary

Acuity   The ability of the visual system to resolve two separate stimuli; "sharpness" of pattern vision.

Amnesia   An impairment of memory that is not secondary to perceptual, attentional, or other cognitive disorders, which can affect memory for events prior to the onset of the amnesia (retrograde) or after (anterograde). When amnesia is caused by brain damage, the affected areas are usually the medial temporal structures (hippocampus and amygdala) or the diencephalon. Such amnesias invariably include an anterograde component; the extent of retrograde amnesia is more variable and very old memories appear always to be spared.

Anomia   An impairment of naming ability that may follow damage to the left hemisphere, and that is not attributable to poor comprehension of what is to be named. Likened by some to the "tip-of-the-tongue" phenomenon that all normal people experience occasionally.

Aphasia   The impairment of language ability following left hemisphere damage, which may affect phonological processing, the comprehension or production of single words, or the use of syntax, usually in differing combinations. The profile of impaired and spared language abilities varies considerably from one aphasic patient to another, depending in part upon the region of the left hemisphere that has been damaged.

Apperceptive agnosia   Broad definition: Any agnosia in which perceptual impairments seem clearly at fault. Narrow definition: A form of visual agnosia in which patients cannot reliably name, match or discriminate even simple geometric shapes, despite adequate visual fields, acuity, and color vision.

Associative agnosia   Broad definition: Any of a number of conditions in which patients cannot name a seen object, despite the absence of gross visual impairments. Narrow definition: A form of visual agnosia in which patients cannot indicate their recognition of a seen object either verbally or nonverbally, despite perceptual abilities adequate for drawing or matching pictures of the object (albeit slowly and in a line-by-line manner).

Basic object level category   Categories that are as general as possible while still maintaining high inter-item similarity. Examples are "chair" (as opposed to "furniture" or "rocking chair") and "apple" (as opposed to "fruit" or "golden delicious apple"). Such categories appear to have some psychological primacy, in that people can generally name or sort stimuli at the basic object level faster than at more general or more specific levels, and children learn the names of basic object level categories before those of other levels.

Confabulation   A false story told by a patient to fill in a gap in memory or insight about his or her situation.

Constructional apraxia   A very general term, denoting an inability to draw (either from memory or by copying) or to assemble the parts of an object.

CT scan   Computerized tomography. An X-ray technique in which the density of tissue can be measured in three dimensions, allowing a fairly high resolution picture of multiple "slices" of the brain.

Disconnection syndrome   A syndrome in which the patient's behavior results from a neuroanatomic disconnection between intact processing centers rather than from a loss of some processing center.

Distributed representation   A way of implementing representations in units of hardware such that the entire set of units is used to represent the entire set of things being represented, by representing each thing as a distinctive pattern of activity across the set of units. This is to be contrasted with local representations, described below.

Dorsal simultanagnosia   An inability to detect more than one object at a time, with difficulty shifting attention from object to object, which generally follows bilateral parieto-occipital damage.

Dorsal visual system   The stream of cortical visual processing going from the occipital to the parietal lobes, concerned with representing spatial locations of stimuli (in contrast to the ventral visual system which is primarily concerned with representing the identity of stimuli). See also Parietal lobe.

Double dissociation   Two abilities are doubly dissociated if each one can be impaired without impairment in the other. Such a dissociation suggests that different underlying psychological processes may be required for the two abilities. In contrast, a single dissociation (i.e., one ability impaired and the other spared) is compatible with the possibility that the same psychological processes underlie the two abilities, but that the impaired ability simply taxes those processes more heavily.

Electroencephalogram (EEG)   A record of the brain's electrical activity recorded from electrodes on the scalp. Abnormalities in the EEG may suggest the nature and rough localization of brain dysfunction.

Event-related potential (ERP)   ERP's are derived from the EEG by averaging intervals of scalp-recorded electrical activity following the presentation of stimuli. The resultant average waveforms contain peaks and troughs whose amplitude and latency are related to different aspects of the processing of the stimulus (e.g., sensory processing, expectancy).

Feature integration   The process of conjoining the separately perceived features of an object (such as color, line orientation) together with one another, to produce the percept of a whole object.

Form from motion   The extraction of shape information from the correlated nature of the movement of the parts of an object. In computerized displays of random dots in which the subsets of the dots move as if they were attached to a rigid moving object, one can experience a strong percept of a solid object of definite size and shape.

Fovea   The central portion of the retina, corresponding to approximately two degrees of visual angle, where acuity is greatest.

Grey matter   Brain tissue comprised primarily of cell bodies (as opposed to axons).

Letter-by-letter reading   A reading strategy adopted by pure alexics, in which words are read by first reading their letters one at a time (either aloud or silently), and then recognizing what word has just been spelled.

Local representation   A way of implementing representations in units of hardware such that each unit is used to represent just one thing, and there is a one-to-one mapping between units and what they represent. This is to be contrasted with distributed representations, described above.

Massively parallel constraint satisfaction   A type of computation in which representations, consisting of patterns of activation over a large number of interconnected units, are transformed in accordance with the "constraints" on each unit's activation level imposed by the activation level of the other units to which it is connected and the strengths of those connections. The representation that results from such a computation therefore depends upon the starting pattern of activity and the pattern of connection strengths. By adjusting the pattern of connection strengths, the network of units can learn to associate representations with one another (e.g., given one representation, it can produce the other).

Module   Although different authors have proposed different technical meanings for this term, most usages are consistent with the following: An information-processing component of the mind which is dedicated to one particular ability (e.g., face recognition), and the internal workings of which are functionally independent from other information-processing mechanisms (i.e., a module will get its input from other mechanisms, but will not "consult" them in the process of formulating its output). As a general view of mental architecture, "modularity" is often contrasted with "unified architectures," according to which our many different cognitive abilities emerge from a relatively limited, common set of basic information-processing mechanisms.

Neurological signs   Objective evidence of neurological abnormality gathered in the course of a physical examination. Excludes subjective symptoms (e.g., headache) that can only be reported by the patient.

Object-centered representation   A representation of object shape in which the locations of the parts are specified with respect to a frame of reference intrinsic to the object (e.g., with respect to the object's own top, bottom, front, back, left, and right).

Occipital lobe   A region of the brain exclusively concerned with vision, and containing primary visual cortex (i.e., the first cortical area to which visual signals are relayed). Figure 33 shows the location of the occipital lobes at the back of the brain.

Optic aphasia   A condition in which patients can (1) name an object if it is presented nonvisually (e.g., by hearing a definition of the object), (2) demonstrate their recognition of the object if it is presented visually (e.g., make an appropriate pantomime showing the use of the object), but (3) cannot name the object when presented visually.

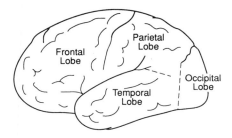

Figure 33
Lateral view of a left hemisphere showing the locations of the 4 lobes.

Parallel distributed processing   See Massively parallel constraint satisfaction.

Parietal lobe   A region of the brain concerned primarily with tactile (anterior parietal cortex) and visual processing, the parietal lobe is particularly important for the "spatial" aspects of vision. Lesions produce impairments in learning spatial locations of stimuli, reaching for visual stimuli, and allocating attention to stimuli in contralesional locations. Figure 33 shows the location of the parietal lobes.

Perceptual categorization   Our ability to recognize the equivalence of many different possible images of an object under different viewing angles, conditions of illumination, and so forth.

Perseveration   The repeating of a response on subsequent trials when it is no longer correct.

Prosopagnosia   The inability to recognize faces, despite generally intact visual perception and the ability to recognize most other types of objects.

Pure alexia   A selective impairment in reading, with normal writing and aural language comprehension. When pure alexics can read at all, they do so letter by letter.

Scotoma   A small visual field defect or blind spot caused by localized damage to the visual cortex or fibers projecting to it.

Semantic knowledge   A frankly vague term referring to our sum total knowledge of the world in general, excluding information that is particular to our own experience (e.g., what we ate for breakfast this morning).

Simultanagnosia   A term that has been applied to a wide variety of different kinds of patients, whose perception of the individual parts of a complex visual display is better than the perception of the whole. See also Dorsal simultanagnosia and Ventral simultanagnosia.

Single unit recording   A technique for monitoring brain activity in animals, in which a microelectrode is placed inside the brain, and the responses of a single cell to different stimuli are recorded.

Skin conductance response   The change in skin conductance, measured by electrodes attached to the hand or some other accessible body part, in response to a stimulus. The SCR is a measure of autonomic arousal, and is sensitive to the degree of psychological "significance" a stimulus has for a subject.

Stroke   The sudden onset of a neurological deficit caused by cerebrovascular disease, most commonly the interruption of blood flow to the brain as a result of blockage of an artery or bleeding into the brain.

Structural description   A kind of shape representation in which a relatively complex shape is described in terms of relatively simpler parts and the relations among the parts.

Syndrome   A set of signs and symptoms that co-occur.

Tachistoscope   A device for presenting visual stimuli for brief and precisely measured amounts of time.

Temporal lobe   A region of the brain with many functions, including audition, memory, language (on the left), and vision. On the basis of single-unit recording and lesion studies in monkeys, as well as neuropsychological studies of brain-damaged humans, the inferior surface of the temporal lobe ("inferotemporal cortex") seems particularly important for object recognition. A population of neurons that respond selectively to faces has recently been found in the superior temporal sulcus of monkeys, a region of temporal cortex further up and on the lateral side of the temporal lobe. Figure 33 shows the location of the temporal lobe.

Top-down processing   This refers to the influence of later stages of processing on earlier stages. For example, word recognition is generally viewed as a later stage of visual perception than letter recognition. Thus if the lexical status (word or nonword) of a letter string affects the recognition of the individual letters in it, this is a case of top-down processing.

Ventral simultanagnosia   A reduction in the ability to rapidly recognize multiple visual stimuli, such that recognition proceeds part by part (i.e., letter-by-letter for words, object-by-object or feature-by-feature for complex nonverbal stimuli). Generally follows left inferior temporo-occipital damage.

Ventral visual system   The stream of cortical visual processing going from the occipital to the temporal lobes, concerned primarily with representing the identity of stimuli by such visual characteristics as shape and color (in contrast to the dorsal visual system, which is primarily concerned with representing the spatial location of stimuli). See also Temporal lobe.

Visual fields   The region of visual space that can be seen without moving the eyes. Brain lesions can cause areas of blindness, known as "visual field defects" either by damage to the visual cortex of the occipital lobe or by interruption of the nerve fibers carrying visual information from the eyes to the visual cortex. If the entire visual cortex of one hemisphere (or the pathways to it) is destroyed, there is blindness on the opposite side of space, known as a homonymous hemianopia. Sometimes only a quarter of the visual field will be impaired because of the way in which the optic pathways fan out on their way to the visual cortices of each hemisphere, in which case the visual field defect is termed a "quadrantanopia."

Visual imagery   The calling up of an image of something in the "mind's eye," which seems to involve the top-down activation of stimulus representations in the visual system.

Visual neglect   A disorder of attention that most commonly follows posterior parietal lobe damage. Although patients with neglect may be capable of responding to a visual stimulus in the contralesional hemifield if there are no competing stimuli elsewhere in the visual field, under normal viewing conditions they appear not to see contralesional stimuli.

White matter   Brain tissue dense in axons, and therefore important for communication between different cortical areas.

Word forms   The groupings of letters in words, corresponding to the orthography of entire words or portions of words.

Word superiority effect   The finding that an individual letter is perceived more quickly and accurately when embedded in a word than in a nonword letter string.

References

Adler, A. (1944). Disintegration and restoration of optic recognition in visual agnosia: Analysis of a case. *Archives of Neurology and Psychiatry*, 51, 243–259.

Aimard, G., Vighetto, A., Confavreux, C., and Devic, M. (1981). La desorientation spatiale. *Revue Neurologique*, 137, 97–111.

Albert, M. L., Reches, A., and Silverberg, R. (1975). Associative visual agnosia without alexia. *Neurology*, 25, 322–326.

Albert, M. L., Soffer, D., Silverberg, R., Reches, A. (1979). The anatomic basis of visual agnosia. *Neurology*, 29, 876–879.

Alexander, M. P., and Albert, M. L. (1983). The anatomical basis of visual agnosia. In A. Kertesz (Ed.), *Localization in Neuropsychology*. New York: Academic Press.

Allport, D. A. (1980). Patterns and actions: Cognitive mechanisms are content-specific. In G. Claxton (Ed.), *Cognitive psychology: New directions*. London: Routledge and Kegan Paul.

Andersen, R. A. (1989). Visual and eye movement functions of the posterior parietal cortex. *Annual Review of Neuroscience*, 12, 377–403.

Anderson, J. R. (1976). Language, memory, and thought. Hillsdale, NJ: Lawrence Erlbaum Associates.

Aptman, M., Levin, H., and Senelick, R. C. (1977). Alexia without agraphia in a left-handed patient with prosopagnosia. *Neurology*, 27, 533–537.

Assal, G. (1969). Regression des troubles de la reconnaissance des physionomes et de la memoire topographique chez un malade opere d'un hematome intracerebral parieto-temporal droit. *Revue Neurologique*, 121, 184–185.

Assal, G. Favre, C., and Anderes, J. (1984). Nonrecognition of familiar animals by a farmer: Zooagnosia or prosopagnosia for animals. *Revue Neurolologique*, 140, 580–584.

Assal, G., and Regli, F. (1980). Syndrome de disconnection visuo-verbale et visuo-gesturelle. *Revue Neurologique*, 136, 365–376.

Baddeley, A. D. (1964). Immediate memory and the perception of letter sequences. *Quarterly Journal of Experimental Psychology*, 16, 364–368.

Bauer, R. M. (1982). Visual hypoemotionality as a symptom of visual-limbic disconnection in man. *Archives of Neurology*, 39, 702–708.

Bauer, R. M. (1984). Autonomic recognition of names and faces in prosopagnosia: A neuropsychological application of the guilty knowledge test. *Neuropsychologia*, 22, 457–469.

Bauer, R. M., and Rubens, A. B. (1985). Agnosia. In K. M. Heilman and E. Valenstein (Ed.), *Clinical Neuropsychology*. New York: Oxford University Press.2nd edition.

Bauer, R. M., and Trobe, J. D. (1984). Visual memory and perceptual impairments in prosopagnosia. *Journal of Clinical Neuro-opthalmology*, 4, 39–46.

Bauer, R. M., and Verfaellie, M. (1988). Electrodermaldiscrimination of familiar but not unfamiliar faces in prosopagnosia. *Brain and Cognition*, 8, 240–252.

Bay, E. (1953). Disturbances of visual perception and their examination. Brain, 76, 515–530.

Baylis, G. C., Rolls, E. T., and Leonard, C. M. (1985). Selectivity between faces in the responses of a population of neurons in the cortex in the superior temporal sulcus of the monkey. *Brain Research*, 342, 91–102.

Baynes, K., Holtzman, J. D., and Volpe, B. T. (1986). Components of visual attention: Alterations in response pattern to visual stimuli following parietal lobe infarction. *Brain*, 109, 99–114.

Beauvois, M. F. (1982). Optic aphasia: A process of interaction between vision and language. *Philosophical Transactions of the Royal Society*, London, B298, 35–47.

Beauvois, M. F., and Saillant, B. (1985). Optic aphasia for colours and colour agnosia: A distinction between visual and visuo-verbal impairments in the processing of colours. *Cognitive Neuropsychology*, 2, 1–48.

Bender, M. B., and Feldman, M. (1972). The so-called 'visual agnosias'. Brain, 95, 173–186.

Benke, T. (1988). Visual agnosia and amnesia from a left unilateral lesion. *European Neurology*, 28, 236–239.

Benson, D. F. and Greenberg, J. P. (1969). Visual form agnosia. *Archives of Neurology*, 20, 82–89.

Benson, D. F., Segarra, J., and Albert, M. L. (1973). Visual agnosia-prosopagnosia: A clinicopathologic correlation. *Archives of Neurology*, 30, 307–310.

Benton, A. L. (1980). The neuropsychology of face recognition. *American Psychologist*, 35, 176–186.

Benton, A. L., and Van Allen, M. W. (1968). Impairment in facial recognition in patients with cerebral disease. Transactions of the American Neurological Association, 93, 38–42.

Benton, A. L., and Van Allen, M. W. (1972). Prosopagnosia and facial discrimination. *Journal of Neurological Sciences*, 15, 167–172.

Beyn, E. S., Knyazeva, G. R. (1962). The problem of prosopagnosia. Journal of Neurology, *Neurosurgery and Psychiatry*, 25, 154–158.

Biederman, I. (1972). Perceiving real-world scenes. Science, 177, 77–79.

Biederman, I. (1987). Recognition-by-components: A theory of human image understanding. *Psychological Review*, 94, 115–147.

Bisiach, E. (1966). Perceptual factors in the pathogenesis of anomia. Cortex, 2, 90–95.

Bisiach, E., Luzzatti, C., and Perani, D. (1979). Unilateral neglect, representational schema and consciousness. *Brain*, 102, 609–618.

Bornstein, B. (1963). Prosopagnosia. In L. Halpern (Ed.), Problems of Dynamic Neruology. Jerusalem: Hadassah Medical Organization, 283–318.

Bornstein, B., and Kidron, D. P. (1959). Prosopagnosia. *Journal of Neurology, Neurosurgery, and Psychiatry*, 22, 124–131.

Bornstein, B., Stroka, H., and Munitz, H. (1969). Prosopagnosia with animal face agnosia. *Cortex*, 5, 164–169.

Boudouresques, J., Poncet, M., Cherif, A., and Balzamo, M. (1979). L'agnosie de visages: un temoin de la desorganisation fonctionnelle d'un certain type de connaissance des elements du monde exterieur. *Bulletin de l' Academie Nationale de Medicine*, 163, 695–702.

Boudouresques, J., Poncet, M., Sebahoun, M., Alicherif, A. (1972). Two cases of alexia without agraphia with disorders of color and image naming. *Bulletin de l'Academie Nationale de Medicine*, 44, 297–303.

Brown, J. W. (1972). Aphasia, Apraxia and Agnosia: Clinical and Theoretical Aspects. Springfield, IL: Charles C. Thomas.

Bruce, C. (1982). Face recognition by monkeys: Absence of an inversion effect. *Neuropsychologia*, 20, 515–521.

Bruce, V., and Young, A. (1986). Understanding face recognition. *British Journal of Psychology*, 77, 305–327.

Brunn, J. L., and Farah, M. J. (in press). The relation between spatial attention and reading: Evidence from the neglect syndrome. *Cognitive Neuropsychology*.

Bruyer, R., Laterre, C., Seron, X., Feyereisne, P., Strypstein, E., Pierrard, E., Rectem, D. (1983). A case of prosopagnosia with some preserved covert remembrance of familiar faces. *Brain and Cognition*, 2, 257–284.

Bub, D. N., Black, S., and Howell, J. (1989). Word recognition and orthographic context effects in a letter-by-letter reader. *Brain and Language*, 36, 357–376.

Cambier, J., Masson, M., Elghozi, D., Henin, D., Viader, F. (1980). Visual agnosia without right hemianopia in a right-handed patient. *Revue Neurologique*, 136, 727–740.

Campion, J. (1987). Apperceptive agnosia: The specification and description of constructs. In G. W. Humphreys, and M. J. Riddoch (Ed.), Visual Object Processing: A Cognitive Neuropsychological Approach . London: Lawrence Erlbaum Associates.

Campion, J., Latto, R. (1985). Apperceptive agnosia due to carbon monoxide poisoning: An interpretation based on critical band masking from disseminated lesions. *Behavioral Brain Research*, 15, 227–240.

Campion, J., Latto, R., and Smith, Y. M. (1983). Is blindsight an effect of scattered light spared cortex, and near-threshold vision? *The Behavioral and Brain Sciences*, 3, 423–447.

Caplan, L. R., and Hedley-Whyte, T. (1974). Cuing and memory dysfunction in alexia without agraphia. *Brain*, 97, 251–262.

Caramazza, A. (1984). The logic of neuropsychological research and the problem of patient classification in aphasia. *Brain and Language*, 21, 9–20.

Cohn, R., Neumann, M.A., Wood, D.H. (1977). Prosopagnosia: a clinicopathological study. *Annals of Neurology*, 1, 177–182.

Cole, M., and Perez-Cruet, J. (1964). Prosopagnosia. *Neuropsychologia*, 2, 237–246.

Coslett, H. B., Saffran, E. M. (1989). Preserved object recognition and reading comprehension in optic aphasia. *Brain*, 112, 1091–1110.

Critchley, M. (1964). The problem of visual agnosia. *Journal of the Neurological Sciences*, 1, 274–290.

Damasio, A. R. (1985). Disorders of complex visual processing: Agnosia, achromatopsia, Balint's syndrome, and related difficulties of orientation and construction. In Mesulam, M. M. (Ed.), Principles of Behavioral Neurology. Philadelphia, PA: F. A. Davis Company, 259–288.

Damasio, A. R., and Damasio, H. (1983). The anatomic basis of pure alexia. *Neurology*, 33, 1573–1583.

Damasio, A. R., Damasio, H., and Van Hoesen, G. W. (1982). Prosopagnosia: Anatomic basis and behavioral mechanisms. *Neurology*, 32, 331–341.

Davidoff, J., and Wilson, B. (1985). A case of visual agnosia showing a disorder of presemantic vision classification. *Cortex*, 21, 121–134.

De Haan, E. H. F., Young, A., and Newcombe, F. (1987). Faces interfere with name classification in a prosopagnosic patient. *Cortex*, 23, 309–316.

Dejerine, J. (1914). Semiologie des Affections du Systeme Nerveux. Paris: Masson.

Dejerine, J. (1892). Contribution a l'etude anatomoclinique et clinique des differentes varietes de cecite verbale. *Memoires de la Societe de Biologie*, 4, 61–90.

Dennis, M. (1976). Dissociated naming and locating of body parts after left anterior temporal lobe resection: An experimental case study. *Brain and Language*, 3, 147–163.

De Renzi, E. (1982). Disorders of Space Exploration and Cognition. New York: John Wiley and Sons.

De Renzi, E. (1986a). Prosopagnosia in two patients with CT scan evidence of damage confined to the right hemisphere. *Neuropsychologia*, 24, 385–389.

De Renzi, E. (1986b). Current issues in prosopagnosia. In H. D. Ellis, M. A. Jeeves, F. Newcome, and A. Young (Ed.), Aspects of Face Processing . Dordrecht: Martinus Nijhoff.

De Renzi, E., Scotti, G., and Spinnler, H. (1969). Perceptual and associative disorders of visual recognition: Relationship to the side of the cerebral lesion. *Neurology*, 19, 634–642.

Desimone, R., Albright, T. D., Gross, C. D., and Bruce, C. (1984). Stimulus-selective responses of inferior temporal neurons in the macaque. *Journal of Neuroscience*, 4, 2051–2062.

Duara, R., Phatak, P. G., and Wadia, N. H. (1975). Prosopagnosia and associated disorders. *Neurology India*, 23, 149–155.

Dumont, I., Griggio, A., Dupont, H., and Jacquy, J. (1981). A propos d'un cas d'agnosie visuelle avec prosopagnosie et agnosie des coleurs. *Acta Psychiatrica Belgica*, 81, 25–45.

Duncan, J. (1984). Selective attention and the organization of visual information. *Journal of Experimental Psychology: General*, 113, 501–517.

Efron, R. (1968). What is perception? Boston Studies in Philosophy of Science, 4, 137–173.

Ekstrom, R., French, J. W., and Harman, H. H. (1976). Manual for Kit of Factor-Referenced Cognitive Tests. Princeton, NJ: Educational Testing Service.

Ellis, W. D. (1938). A Sourcebook of Gestalt Psychology. New York: Harcourt Brace.

Ellis, A. W., and Young, A. W. (1988). Human Cognitive Neuropsychology. Hillsdale, NJ: Lawrence Erlbaum Associates.

Eriksen, C. W., and Spencer, T. (1969). Rate of information processing in visual perception: Some results and methodological considerations. *Journal of Experimental Psychology Monograph*, Vol. 79.

Etcoff, N. L. (1984). Selective attention to facial identity and facial emotion. *Neuropsychologia*, 22, 281–295.

Ettlinger, G. (1956). Sensory deficits in visual agnosia. *Journal of Neurology, Neurosurgery and Psychiatry*, 19, 297–301.

Farah, M. J. (1988). Is visual imagery really visual? Overlooked evidence from neuropsychology. *Psychological Review*, 95, 307–317.

Farah, M. J. (in press). Patterns of co-occurrence among the associative agnosias: Implications for the nature of visual object representation. *Cognitive Neuropsychology*.

Farah, M. J., Wallace, M. A., Brunn, J. L., and Madigan, N. (1989). Structure of objects in central vision affects the distribution of visual attention in neglect. *Society for Neuroscience Abstracts*, 15, 481.

Farah, M. J., Hammond, K. H., Mehta, Z., and Ratcliff, G. (1989). Category-specificity and modality-specifity in semantic memory. *Neuropsychologia*, 27, 193–200.

Farah, M. J., Wong, A. B., Monheit, M. A., and Morrow, L. A. (1989). Parietal lobe mechanisms of spatial attention: Modality-specific or supramodal? *Neuropsychologia*, 27, 461–470.

Faust, C. (1955). Die zerebralen herdstorungen bein hinterhaupverletzungen und ihre beuteilung. Stuttgart: Verlag.

Feinberg, T. E., Gonzalez-Rothi, L. J., Heilman, K. M. (1986). Multimodal agnosia after unilateral left hemisphere lesion. *Neurology*, 36, 864–867.

Ferro, J. M. and Santos, M. E. (1984). Associative visual agnosia: A case study. *Cortex*, 20, 121–134.

Frederiks, J. A. M. (1969). The agnosias. In P. J. Vinken, and G. W. Bruyn (Eds.), Handbook of Clinical Neurology. Amsterdam: North Holland.

Friedman, R. B., Alexander, M. P. (1984). Pictures, Images, and Pure Alexia: A Case Study. *Cognitive Neuropsychology*, 1, 9–23.

Gelb, A., and Goldstein, K. (1918). Analysis of a case of figural blindness. *Neurology and Psychology*, 41, 1–143.

Geschwind, N. (1965). Disconnexion syndromes in animals and man. Part II. *Brain*, 88, 585–645.

Gibson, J. J. (1979). The Ecological Approach to Visual Perception. Boston: Houghton Mifflin.

Gil, R., Pluchon, C., Toullat, G., Michenau, D., Rogez, R., and Levevre, J. P. (1985). Disconnexion visuo-verbale (aphasie optique) pour les objets, les images, les couleurs et les visages avec alexie 'abstractive'. *Neuropsychologia*, 23, 333–349.

Girotti, F., Milanese, C., Casazza, M., Allegranza, A., Corridori, F., Avanzini, G. (1982). Oculomotor disturbances in Balint's syndrome: Anatomoclinical findings and electrooculographic analysis in a case. *Cortex*, 18, 603–614.

Gloning, I., Gloning, K., Jellinger, K., and Quatember, R. (1970). A case of prosopagnosia with necropsy findings. *Neuropsychologia*, 8, 199–204.

Glowic, C., and Violon, A. (1981). Un cas de prosopagnosie regressive. *Acta Neurologica Belgica*, 81, 86–97.

Godwin-Austen, R. B. (1965). A case of visual disorientation. *Journal of Neurology, Neurosurgery and Psychiatry*, 28, 453–458.

Goldstein, K., and Gelb, A. (1918). Psychologische analysen hirnpathologischer falle auf grund von untersuchungen hirnverletzer. *Zeitschrift fur die gesante Neurologie and Psychiatrie*, 41, 1–142.

Gomori, A. J., and Hawryluk, G. A. (1984). Visual agnosia without alexia. *Neurology*, 34, 947–950.

Greenblatt, S. H. (1983). Localization of lesions in alexia. In A. Kertesz (Ed.), Localization in Neuropsychology . New York: Academic Press.

Guard, O., Graule, A., Spautz, J. M., and Dumas, R. (1981). Anomie fabulante par agnosie visuelle et tactile au cours d'une demence arteriopathique. *L'Encephale*, 7, 275–291.

Hart, J., Berndt, R. S., and Caramazza, A. (1985). Category-specific naming deficit following cerebral infarction. *Nature*, 316, 439–440.

Hecaen, H., and de Ajuriaguerra, J. (1956). Agnosie visuelle pour les objets inanimes par lesion unilaterale gauche. *Revue Neurologique*, 94, 222–233.

Hecaen, H., Goldblum, M. C., Masure, M. C., Ramier, A. M. (1974). A new case of object agnosia. A deficit in association or categorization specific for the visual modality. *Neuropsychologia*, 12, 447–464.

Herman, M., and Kanade, T. (1986). Incremental reconstruction of 3-D scenes from multiple complex images. *Artificial Intelligence*, 30, 289–341.

Hinton, G. E. (1981). A parallel computation that assigns canonical object-based frames of reference. Proceedings of the International Joint Conference on Artificial Intelligence. Vancouver, Canada.

Hinton, G. E., McClelland, J. L., and Rumelhart, D. E. (1986). Distributed Representations. In D. E. Rumelhart, and J. L. McClelland (Ed.), Parallel Distributed Processing: Explorations in the Microstructure of Cognition. Cambridge: The MIT Press.

Holender, D. (1986). Semantic activation without conscious identification in dichotic listening, paratoveal vision, and visual masking. A survey and appraisal. *Behavioral and Brain Sciences*, 9, 1–66.

Holmes, G. (1918). Disturbances of visual orientation. *British Journal of Ophthalmology*, 2, 449–468 and 506–518.

Holmes, G. and Horrax, G. (1919). Disturbances of spatial orientation and visual attention with loss of stereoscopic vision. *Archives of Neurology and Psychiatry*, 1, 385–407.

Humphreys, G. W. and Riddoch, M. J. (1984). Routes to object constancy: Implications from neurological impairments of object constancy. *Quarterly Journal of Experimental Psychology*, 36A, 385–415.

Humphreys, G. W., and Riddoch, M. J. (1985). Author's correction to 'Routes to object constancy'. *Quarterly Journal of Experimental Psychology*, 37A, 493–495.

Humphreys, G. W., and Riddoch, M. J. (1987a). To See but Not to See: A Case Study of Visual Agnosia. Hillsdale, NJ: Lawrence Erlbaum Associates.

Humphreys, G. W., and Riddoch, M. J. (1987b). The fractionation of visual agnosia. In G. W. Humphreys, and M. J. Riddoch (Ed.), Visual Object Processing: A Cognitive Neuropsychological Approach . London: Lawrence Erlbaum Associates.

Ikeuchi, K. (1987). Generating an interpretation tree from a CAD model for 3-D object recognition in bin-picking tasks. International Journal of Computer Vision, 1, 145–165.

Jung, C. (1949). Über eine Nachuntersuchung des Falles Schn. von Goldstein und Gelb. *Psychiatrie, Neurologie und Medizinische Psychologie*, 1, 353–362.

Karpov, B. A., Meerson, Y. A., and Tonkonough, I. M. (1979). On some peculiarities of the visuomotor system in visual agnosia. *Neuropsychologia*, 17, 281–294.

Kase, C. S., Troncoso, J. F., Court, J. E., Tapia, F. J., Mohr, J. P. (1977). Global spatial disorientation. *Journal of the Neurological Sciences*, 34, 267–278.

Kaufman, L. (1974). Sight and mind. New York: Oxford University Press.

Kawahata, N., and Nagata, K. (1989). A case of associative visual agnosia: Neuropsychological findings and theoretical considerations. *Journal of Clinical and Experimental Neuropsychology*, 11, 645–664.

Kay, M. C., and Levin, H. S. (1982). Prosopagnosia. *American Journal of Opthamology*, 94, 75–80.

Kendrick, K. M., and Baldwin, B. A. (1987). Cells in temporal cortex of conscious sheep can respond preferentially to faces. *Science*, 236, 448–450.

Kertesz, A. (1979). Visual agnosia: The dual deficit of perception and recognition. *Cortex*, 15, 403–419.

Kertesz, A. (1987). The clinical spectrum and localization of visual agnosia. In G. W. Humphreys, and M. J. Riddoch (Ed.), Visual Object Processing: A Cognitive Neuropsychological Approach . London: Lawrence Erlbaum Associates.

Kinsbourne, M. and Warrington, E. K. (1962). A disorder of simultaneous form perception. *Brain*, 85, 461–486.

Kinsbourne, M., and Warrington, E. K. (1963). The localizing significance of limited simultaneous form perception. *Brain*, 86, 697–702.

Konorski, J. (1967). Integrative Activity of the Brain. Chicago: University of Chicago Press.

Kosslyn, S. M. (1980). Image and Mind. Cambridge: Harvard University Press.

Kosslyn, S. M. (1987). Seeing and imagining in the cerebral hemispheres: A computational approach. *Psychological Review*, 94, 148–175.

Kosslyn, S., Flynn, R., Amsterdam, J., Wang, G. (in press). Components of high-level vision: A cognitive neuroscience analysis and accounts of neurological syndromes. *Cognition*.

Kumar, N., Verma, A., Maheshwari, M. C., and Kumar, B. R. (1986). Prosopagnosia (A report of two cases). Journal of the Association of Physicians of India, 34, 733–735.

Kurucz, J., and Feldmar, G. (1979). Prosopo-affective agnosia as a symptom of cerebral organic disease. *Journal of American Geriatric Society*, 27, 225–230.

Landis, T., Cummings, J. L., Christen, L., Bogen, J. E., Imhof, H. (1986). Are unilateral right posterior cerebral lesions sufficient to cause prosopagnosia? Clinical and radiological findings in six additional patients. *Cortex*, 22, 243–252.

Landis, T., Graves, R., Benson, F., Hebben, N. (1982). Visual recognition through kinaesthetic mediation. *Psychological Medicine*, 12, 515–531.

Landis, T., Regard, M., Bliestle, A., Kleihues, P. (1988). Prosopagnosia and agnosia for noncanonical views. *Brain*, 111, 1287–1297.

Lapedes, A. S., and Farber, R. (1987). Nonlinear signal processing using neural networks: Prediction and system modeling. Technical Report, Los Alamos National Laboratory.

Larrabee, G. J., Levin, H. S., Huff, F. J., Kay, M. C., and Guinto, F. C. (1985). Visual agnosia contrasted with visual-verbal disconnection. *Neuropsychologia, 23,* 1–12.

Levine, D. N. (1978). Prosopagnosia and visual object agnosia: A behavioral study. *Neuropsychologia, 5,* 341–365.

Levine, D. N., and Calvanio, R. (1978). A study of the visual defect in verbal alexia-simultanagonosia. *Brain,* 101, 65–81.

Levine, D. N., and Calvanio, R. (1982). The neurology of reading disorders. In Arbib, M. A., Caplan, D., and Marshall, J. C. (Ed.), Neural Models of Language Processes . New York: Academic Press.

Levine, D., and Calvanio, R. (1989). Prosopagnosia: A defect in visual configural processing. *Brain and Cognition,* 10, 149–170.

Levin, H. S., and Peters, B. H. (1976). Neuropsychological testing following head injuries: Prosopagnosia without visual field defect. *Diseases of the Nervous System,* 37, 68–71.

Lezak, M. (1983). 2nd Ed.. Neuropsychological assessment. New York: Oxford University Press.

Lhermitte, F., and Beauvois, M. F. (1973). A visual-speech disconnexion syndrome: Report of a case with optic aphasia, agnosic alexia and colour agnosia. Brain, 96, 695–714.

Lhermitte, J., Chain, F., Escourolle, R., Ducarne, B., and Pillon, B. (1972). Etude anatomo-clinque d'un cas de prosopagnosie. *Revue Neurologigue,* 126, 329–346.

Lhermitte, F., Chain, F., Aron-Rosa, D., Leblanc, M., and Souty, O. (1969). Enregistrement des mouvements du regard dans un cas d'agnosie visuelle et dans un cas de desorientation spatiale. *Revue Neurologique,* 121, 121–137.

Lhermitte, F., and Pillon, B. (1975). La prosopagnosie. Role de l'hemisphere droit dans la perception visuelle. *Revue Neurologigue,* 131, 791–812.

Liepmann, H. (1900). Das Krankheitschild der Apraxie. *Monatsschrift fur Psychiatrie und Neurologie,* 8, 15–44, 102–132, 182–197.

Lissauer,H. (1890). Ein fall von seelenblindheit nebst einem Beitrage zur Theori derselben. *Archiv fur Psychiatrie und Nervenkrankheiten,* 21, 222–270.

Lowe, D. G. (1987). The viewpoint consistency constraint. *International Journal of Computer Vision,* 1, 57–72.

Luria, A. R. (1959). Disorders of 'simultaneous perception' in a case of bilateral occipitoparietal brain injury. *Brain,* 83, 437–449.

Luria, A. R. (1973). The Working Brain. New York: Basic Books.

Luria, A. R., Pravdina-Vinarskaya, E. N., and Yarbuss, A. L. (1963). Disorders of ocular movement in a case of simultanagnosia. *Brain,* 86, 219–228.

Mack, J. L., and Boller, F. (1977). Associative visual agnosia and its related deficits: the role of the minor hemisphere in assigning meaning to visual perceptions. *Neuropsychologia,* 15, 345–349.

Macrae, D., and Trolle, E. (1956). The defect of function in visual agnosia. Brain, 79, 94–110.

Malone, D. R., Morris, H. H., Kay, M. C., and Levin, S. H. (1982). Prosopagnosia: a double dissociation between the recognition of familiar and unfamiliar faces. *Journal of Neurology, Neurosurgery, and Psychiatry,* 45, 820–822.

Marcel, A. J. (1983). Conscious and unconscious perception: Experiments on visual masking and word recognition. *Cognitive Psychology,* 15, 197–237.

Marks, R. L., and De Vito, T. (1987). Alexia without agraphia and associated disorders: Importance of recognition in the rehabilitation setting. *Archives of Physical Medicine and Rehabilitation,* 68, 239–243.

Marr, D. (1982). Vision. San Francisco: Freeman.

Marr, D., and Nishihara, H. K. (1978). Representation and recognition of the spatial organization of three-dimensional shapes. *Proceedings of the Royal Society of London*, B200, 269–294.

Marx, P., Boquet, J., Luce, R., Farbos, J.P. (1970). Spatial agnosia and agnosia of physiogomies, sequelae of cortical blindness. *Bulletin des Societes d'Ophtalmologie*, Vol. 70.

McCarthy, R.A., Warrington, E.K. (1986). Visual associative agnosia: a clinico-anatomical study of a single case. *Journal of Neurology, Neurosurgery, and Psychiatry*, 49, 1233–1240.

McCleary, C., and Hirst, W. (1986). Semantic classification in aphasia: A study of basic, superordinate, and function relations. *Brain and Language*, 27, 199–109.

McClelland, J. L., Rumelhart, D. E. (1981). An interactive activation model of context effects in letter perception: Part 1. An account of basic findings. *Psychological Review*, 88, 375–407.

McClelland, J. L., Rumelhart, D. E. and Hinton, G. E. (1986). The appeal of parallel distributed processing. In Rumelhart, D. E and McClelland, J. L. (Ed.), Parallel Distributed Processing: Explorations in the Microstructure of Cognition . Cambridge, MA: The MIT Press.

Meadows, J. C. (1974). The anatomical basis of prosopagnosia. *Journal of Neurology, Neurosurgery, and Psychiatry*, 37, 489–501.

Mendez, M. F. (1988). Visuoperceptual function in visual agnosia. *Neurology*, 38, 1754–1759.

Mesulam, M. M. (1985). Patterns in behavioral neuroanatomy. In Mesulam, M. M. (Ed.), Principles of Behavioral Neurology. Philadelphia, PA: F. A. Davis Company, 1–70.

Michel, F., Perenin, M. T., and Sieroff, E. (1986). Prosopagnosie sans hemianopsie apres lesion unilaterale occipito-temporale droite. *Revue Neurologique*, 142, 545–549.

Michimata, C., and Hellige, J. B. (1987). Effects of blurring and stimulus size on the lateralized processing of nonverbal stimuli. *Neuropsychologia*, 25, 397–407.

Morin, P., Rivrain, Y., Eustache, F., Lambert, J., and Courtheoux, P. (1984). Agnosie visuelle et agnosie tactile. *Revue Neurologique*, 140, 271–277.

Morrow, L. A., and Ratcliff, G. (1988). The disengagement of covert attention and the neglect syndrome. *Psychobiology*, 3, 16, 261–269.

Mouren, P., Tatossian, A., Trupheme, R., Giudicelli, S., and Fresco, R. (1967). L'alexie par deconnection visuo-verbale (Geschwind): A propos d'un das de cecite verbale pure sans agraphie avec troubles de la denomination des couleurs, des nombres et des images. *Encephale*, 56, 112–137.

Muller, H. J. and Findlay, J. M. (1987). Sensitivity and criterion effects in the spatial cuing of visual attention. *Perception & Psychophysics*, 42, 383–399.

Nardelli, E., Buonanno, F., Coccia, G., Fiaschi, H., Terzian, H., and Rizzuto, N. (1982). Prosopagnosia: Report of four cases. *European Neurology*, 21, 289–297.

Neisser, U. (1967). Cognitive Psychology. New York: Appleton-Century-Crofts.

Neville, H. J., and Lawson, D. (1987). Attention to central and peripheral visual space in a movement detection task: An event-related potential and behavioral study. I. Normal hearing adults. *Brain Research*, 405, 253–267.

Newcombe, F. (1979). The processing of visual information in prosopagnosia and acquired dyslexia: Functional versus physiological interpretation. In D. J. Oborne, M. M. Gruneberg, and J. R. Eiser (Ed.), Research in Psychology and Medicine . London: Academic Press.

Newcombe, F. and Ratcliff, G. (1974). Agnosia: A disorder of object recognition. In F. Michel and B. Schott (Eds.), Les Syndromes de Disconnexion Calleuse chez l'Homme. Lyon: Colloque International.

Newcombe, F., Young, A. W. and de Haan, E. H. F. (1989). Prosopagnosia and object agnosia without covert recognition. *Neuropsychologia*, 27, 179–191.

Nielsen, J. M. (1936). Agnosia, Apraxia, and Aphasia: Their Value in Cerebral Localization. New York: Paul Hoeber.

Nielsen, J. M. (1937). Unilateral cerebral dominance as related to mind blindness. *Archives of Neurology and Psychiatry*, 38, 108–135.

Noel, G., and Meyers, C. (1971). Two cases of visual agnosia with achromatognosia. *Acta Neurologica Belgica*, 71, 173–184.

Orgogozo, J. M., Pere, J. J., and Strube, E. (1979). Alexie sans agraphie, 'agnosie' des couleurs et atteinte de l'hemichamp visual droit: Un syndrome de l'artere cerebrale posterieure. Semaines des Hopitaux de Paris, 55, 1389–1394.

Paivio, A. (1971). Imagery and Verbal Processes. New York: Holt, Rinehart, and Winston.

Pallis, C. A. (1955). Impaired identification of faces and places with agnosia for colors. *Journal of Neurology, Neurosurgery and Psychiatry*, 18, 218–224.

Palmer, S. E. (1975). The effects of contextual scenes on the identification of objects. *Memory & Cognition*, 3, 519–526.

Pashler, H., and Badgio, P. (1985). Visual attention and stimulus identification. *Journal of Experimental Psychology: Human Perception and Performance*, 11, 105–121.

Pashler, H., Badgio, P. C. (1987). Attentional issues in the identification of alphanumeric characters. Attention and Performance, Volume XII Lawrence Erlbaum Associates.

Patterson, K. E., and Kay, J. (1982). Letter-by-letter reading: Psychological descriptions of a neurological syndrome. *Quarterly Journal of Experimental Psychology*, 34A, 411–441.

Perrett, D., Rolls, E. T., and Caan, W. (1982). Visual neurons responsive to faces in the monkey temporal cortex. *Experimental Brain Research*, 47, 329–342.

Pillon, B., Signoret, J. L., and Lhermitte, F. (1981). Agnosie visuelle associative: Role de l'hemisphere gauche dans la perception visuelle. Revue Neurologique, 137, 831–842.

Pinker, S. (1985). Visual cognition: An introduction. In S. Pinker (Ed.), Visual Cognition. Cambridge: The MIT Press.

Poeck, K. (1984). Neuropsychological demonstration of splenial interhemispheric disconnection in a case of optic anomia. *Neuropsychologia*, 22, 707–713.

Posner, M. I. (1980). Orienting of attention. *Quarterly Journal of Experimental Psychology*, 32, 3–25.

Posner, M. I., Snyder, C. R. R., and Davidson, B. J. (1980). Attention and the detection of signals. *Journal of Experimental Psychology: General*, 109, 160–174.

Posner, M. I., Walker, J. A., Friedrich, F. J., and Rafal, R. D. (1984). Effects of parietal lobe injury on covert orienting of visual attention. Journal of Neuroscience, 4, 1863–1874.

Pylyshyn, Z. W. (1984). Computation and cognition. Cambridge, MA: MIT Press.

Raizada, V. N., Raizada, I. N. (1972). Visual agnosia. Neurology India, 20, 181–182.

Ratcliff, G., and Newcombe, F. (1982). Object recognition: Some deductions from the clinical evidence. In A. W. Ellis (Ed.), Normality and pathology in cognitive functions. New York: Academic Press.

Reicher, G. M. (1969). Perceptual recognition as a function of meaningfulness of stimulus material. *Journal of Experimental Psychology*, 81, 275–280.

Renault, B., Signoret, J. L., Debruille, B., Breton, F., and Bolgert, F. (1989). Brain potentials reveal covert facial recognition in prosopagnosia. *Neuropsychologia*, 27, 905–912.

Riddoch, M. J., and Humphreys, G. W. (1987a). A case of integrative visual agnosia. *Brain*, 110, 1431–1462.

Riddoch, M. J., and Humphreys, G. W. (1987b). Visual object processing in optic aphasia: a case of semantic access agnosia. *Cognitive Neuropsychology*, 4, 131–185.

Rizzo, M., and Hurtig, R. (1987). Looking but not seeing: Attention, perception, and eye movements in simultanagnosia. *Neurology*, 37, 1642–1648.

Rolls, E. T. (1984). Neurons in the temporal lobe and amygdala of the monkey with responses selective for faces. *Human Neurobiology*, 3, 209–222.

Rolls, E. T., and Baylis, G. C. (1986). Size and contrast have only small effects on the responses to faces of neurons in the cortex of the superior temporal sulcus of the monkey. *Experimental Brain Research*, 65, 38–48.

Rondot, P., Tzavaras, A., and Garcin, R. (1967). Sur un cas de prosopagnosie persistant depuis quinze ans. *Revue Neurologique*, 117, 424–428.

Rosch, E., Mervis, C. B., Gray, W., Johnson, D., and Boyes-Braem, P. (1976). Basic objects in natural categories. *Cognitive Psychology*, 8, 382–439.

Ross, E. D. (1980). Sensory-specific and fractional disorders of recent memory in man: I: Isolated loss of visual recent memory. *Archives of Neurology*, 37, 193–200.

Rouzaud, M., Ribadeau, J. L., Degiovanni, E., Larmande, P., Ployet, M. J., and Laffont, F. (1978). Troubles associatifs visuels (agnosie et syndrome de dysconnexion); atteinte auditive d'origine ischemique. *Revue Otoneuroophtalmologique*, 50, 365–382.

Rubens, A. B., and Benson, D. F. (1971). Associative visual agnosia. *Archives of Neurology*, 24, 305–316.

Schwartz, M. F., Saffran, E. M., and Marin, O. S. M. (1980). Fractionating the reading process in dementia: Evidence for word-specific print-to-sound associations. In M. Coltheart, K. E. Patterson and J. C. Marshall (Ed.), Deep Dyslexia . London: Routledge and Kegan Paul.

Sergent, J., and Hellige, J. B. (1986). Role of input factors in visual field asymmetries. *Brain and Cognition*, 5, 174–199.

Shallice, T. (1988). From Neuropsychology to Mental Structure. New York: Cambridge University Press.

Shaw, M. L. (1984). Division of attention between spatial locations: A fundamental difference between detection of letters and detection of luminance increments. In H. Bouma and D.G. Brouwhuis (Ed.), Attention and Performance X. Hillsdale, NJ: Lawrence Erlbaum Associates, 109–121.

Shepard, R. N. (1978). The mental image. *American Psychologist*, 33, 125–137. (b).

Shiffrin, R. M., and Gardner, G. T. (1972). Visual processing capacity and attentional control. *Journal of Experimental Psychology*, 93, 72–83.

Shuttleworth, E. C., Syring, V., and Allen, N. (1982). Further observations on the nature of prosopagnosia. *Brain and Cognition*, 1, 302–332.

Skinner, B. F. (1965). Science and Human Behavior. New York: Macmillan.

Spreen, O., Benton, A. L., and Van Allen, M. W. (1966). Dissociation of visual and tactile naming in amnesic aphasia. *Neurology*, 16, 807–814.

Squire, L. R. (1987). Memory and Brain. New York: Oxford University Press.

Striano, S., Grossi, D., Chiacchio, and Fels, A. (1981). Bilateral lesion of the occipital lobes. *Acta Neurologica* (Napoli), 36, 690–694.

Taylor, A. M., and Warrington, E. K. (1971). Visual agnosia: a single case report. *Cortex*, 7, 152–161.

Tenenbaum, J. M., and Barrow, H. G. (1976). Experiments in interpretation-guided segmentation. Stanford Research Institiute Technical Note 123.

Teuber, H. L. (1968). Alteration of perception and memory in man. In L. Weiskrantz (Ed.), Analysis of Behavioral Change. New York: Harper and Row.

Theios, J., and Amrhein, P. C. (1989). Theoretical analysis of the cognitive processing of lexical and pictorial stimuli: Reading, naming, and visual and conceptual comparisons. *Psychological Review*, 96, 5–24.

Tranel, D., and Damasio, A. R. (1985). Knowledge without awareness: an autonomic index of facial recognition by prosopagnosics. *Science*, 228, 1453–1454.

Tranel, D., and Damasio, A. R. (1988). Non-conscious face recognition in patients with face agnosia. *Behavioral Brain Research*, 30, 235–249.

Tranel, D., Damasio, A. R., and Damasio, H. (1988). Intact recognition of facial expression, gender, and age in patients with impaired recognition of face identity. *Neurology*, 38, 690–696.

Treisman, A., and Gelade, G. (1980). A feature-integration theory of attention. *Cognitive Psychology*, 12, 97–136.

Tyler, H. R. (1968). Abnormalities of perception with defective eye movements (Balint's syndrome). *Cortex*, 3, 154–171.

Tzavaras, A., Merienne, L., and Masure, M.C. (1973). Prosopagnosie, amnesie et troubles du langage par lesion temporale gauche chez un sujet Gaucher. *Encephale*, 62, 382–394.

Ungerleider, L. G., and Mishkin, M. (1982). Two cortical visual systems. In D. J. Ingle, M. A. Goodale, R. J. W. Mansfield (Ed.), Analysis of Visual Behavior . Cambridge: The MIT Press.

Von Monakow, C. (1914). Die Lokalisation im Grosshirn und der Abbau der Funktion durch Corticale Herde. Wiesbaden: J. F. Bergmann.

Wapner, W., Judd, T., and Gardner, H. (1978). Visual agnosia in an artist. *Cortex*, 14, 343–364.

Warrington, E. K. (1975). The selective impairment of semantic memory. *Quarterly Journal of Experimental Psychology*, 27, 635–657.

Warrington, E. K. (1982). Neuropsychological studies of object recognition. *Philosophical Transactions of the Royal Society* (London), B298, 15–33.

Warrington, E. K. (1985). Agnosia: The impairment of object recognition. In P. J. Vinken, G. W. Bruyn, and H. L. Klawans (Ed.), Handbook of Clinical Neurology. Amsterdam: Elsevier.

Warrington, E. K., and James, M. (1967). An experimental investigation of facial recognition in patients with unilateral cerebral lesions. *Cortex*, 3, 317–326.

Warrington, E. K., and James, M. (1986). Visual object recognition in patients with right-hemisphere lesions: axes or features. *Perception*, 15, 355–366.

Warrington, E. K., and McCarthy, R. (1983). Category specific access dysphasia. *Brain*, 106, 859–878.

Warrington, E. K., and McCarthy, R. (1987). Categories of knowledge: Further fractionation and an attempted integration. *Brain*, 110, 1273–1296.

Warrington, E. K., and Rabin, P. (1971). Visual span of apprehension in patients with unilateral cerebral lesions. *Quarterly Journal of Experimental Psychology*, 23, 423–431.

Warrington, E. K., and Shallice, T. (1980). Word-form dyslexia. *Brain*, 103, 99–112.

Warrington, E. K., and Shallice, T. (1984). Category specific semantic impairments. *Brain*, 107, 829–854.

Warrington, E. K. and Taylor, A. M. (1973). The contribution of the right parietal lobe to visual object recognition. *Cortex*, 9, 152–164.

Warrington, E. K., and Taylor, A. M. (1978). Two categorical stages of object recognition. *Perception*, 7, 695–705.

Wechsler, D. (1981). WAIS-R Manual. New York: Psychological Corporation.

Weiskrantz, L. (1986). Blindsight: A Case Study and Implications. Oxford: Oxford University Press.

Weisstein M., and Harris, C. S. (1974). Visual detection of line segments: An object superiority effect. *Science*, 186, 752–755.

Wheeler, D. D. (1970). Processes in word recognition. *Cognitive Psychology*, 1, 59–85.

Whitely, A. M., and Warrington, E. K. (1977). Prosopagnosia: A clinical, psychological, and anatomical study of three patients. *Journal of Neurology Neurosurgery and Psychiatry*, 40, 395–403.

Williams, M. (1970). Brain Damage and the Mind. Baltimore: Penguin Books.

Wolpert, I. (1924). Die simultanagnosie: Storung der Gesamtauffassung. *Zeitschrift fur die gesante Neurologie and Psychiatrie*, 93, 397–415.

Yamadori, A., and Albert, M. L. (1973). Word category aphasia. Cortex, 9, 112–115.

Yin, R.K. (1969). Looking at upside down faces. *Journal of Experimental Psychology*, 81, 141–145.

Young, A. W. (1987). Finding the mind's construction in the face. *Cognitive Neuropsychology*, 4, 45–53.

Young, A. W. (1988). Functional organization of visual recognition. In L. Weiskrantz (Ed.), Thought Without Language . Oxford: Oxford University Press.

Young, A., and De Haan, E. H. F. (1988). Boundaries of covert recognition in prosopagnosia. *Cognitive Neuropsychology*, 5, 317–336.

Zaidel, E. (1985). Language in the right hemisphere. In D.F. Benson and E. Zaidel (Ed.), The Dual Brain. New York: The Guilford Press, 205–231.

Afterword

About five years ago I sat down at my computer to write the concluding paragraph for *Visual Agnosia*. As I begin this Afterword to the paperback edition, I am cheered by the field's progress in the intervening five years in understanding the neural bases of human object recognition. Continued work in many laboratories with agnosic and normal subjects as well as advances in the use of neuroimaging methods and computational modeling, have all contributed to this progress. In addition to being encouraged by these developments, I am also mightily relieved that none of them has yet rendered obsolete the ideas and findings described in *Visual Agnosia!* Rather, additional converging evidence is now available for some of the conclusions offered within, and the growth of computational neuropsychology has demonstrated in a concrete way the usefulness of connectionist principles for thinking about agnosia.

For readers who would like to follow their reading of this book with a few relevant articles of a more recent vintage, I will make some recommendations here. These references were chosen for their relevance to the issues and framework discussed in the book, and my own work is therefore heavily represented.

The localization of face and object recognition has benefited from the advent of PET activation studies of normal subjects, as well as continued research with focally brain-damaged patients, and these different methodologies yield pleasingly consistent results. Haxby, Grady, Horowitz, Ungerleider, Mishkin, Carson, Herscovitch, Shapiro, and Rapoport (1991) and Sergent, Ohta, and MacDonald (1992) used a variety of face perception tasks with PET and report bilateral fusiform activation, more extensive on the right side. This localization is consistent with the conclusion offered in section 4.2, on the basis of lesions in prosopagnosic patients, but provides a more specific localization than was possible with the available case material. De Renzi, Perani, Carlesimo, Silveri, and Fazio (1994) drew on evidence from brain-damaged patients to address the issue of whether unilateral lesions can cause prosopagnosia and, by implication, the issue of how strongly lateralized face recognition is. They concluded that the functional asymmetry is sufficiently weak in most individuals that left hemisphere mechanisms can suffice following right hemisphere damage, but that for some strongly asymmetrical individuals a single right hemisphere lesion will cause prosopagnosia. Sergent, Zuck, Levesque, and MacDonald (1992) studied object recognition with PET and found left lingual and fusiform activation, consistent with the suggestion made in section 5.5 that unilateral left posterior lesions can cause associative object agnosia without prosopagnosia. Feinberg, Schindler, Ochoa, Kwan, and Farah (in press) specified the critical lesion site for this form of agnosia more precisely by superimposing lesions from a series of cases, concluding that the left parahippocampal, lingual, and fusiform gyri are critical for object and word, but not face, recognition.

One of the central theoretical issues concerning prosopagnosia is whether it is truly selective for faces, or whether recognition of all objects is equally affected but only the most complex objects, namely faces, present any practical difficulty. This is relevant to the question of whether normal humans have special-purpose pattern recognition systems, or only a single general-purpose system. It was surprising to me that by 1990 there had been no direct test of these competing hypotheses and in section 5.2 I was forced to reason on the basis of fairly indirect evidence that face recognition was disproportionately impaired in prosopagnosia. Happily, there are now a few studies that address the issue head on and all conclude that prosopagnosics are more impaired in face recognition than in the recognition of other complex or confusable objects (Farah, Levinson, and Klein, in press; Farah, Wilson, Drain, and Tanaka, in press; McNeill and Warrington, 1993). The conjecture in section 5.5 concerning *how* face recognition differs from object recognition, namely by a relative lack of part decomposition, has found good support in studies conducted with Jim Tanaka (Tanaka and Farah, 1993; Farah, Tanaka, and Drain, in press).

Another issue raised in connection with face recognition in section 4.2 was the mechanism underlying covert recognition of faces in prosopagnosia. Three recent papers have made explicit proposals concerning mechanism: Burton, Young, Bruce, Johnston, and Ellis (1991), De Haan, Bauer, and Greve (1992), and Farah, O'Reilly, and Vecera (1993). The first two differ from the third on the issue of whether covert recognition of faces reflects a true dissociation between normal visual face recognition and conscious awareness, or whether it is the product of a damaged, but not obliterated, face recognition system. Our computer simulation suggests that the tasks used to measure covert recognition are indeed more sensitive to the residual knowledge in a damaged network, as suggested earlier.

The relation between prosopagnosia and problems recognizing living things remains puzzling. On the one hand, these problems are highly associated, and it seems natural to think of faces and living things as belonging together. On the other hand, the problems are not invariably associated, and the impairment with living things in prosopagnosic patients frequently encompasses semantic knowledge as well as visual recognition. The issue is further clouded by the possibility that impairments with living things may not be real at all, but instead result from the greater average difficulty of recognizing living relative to nonliving things. Recent attempts to sort these matters out can be found in Farah, McMullen, and Meyer (1991), Farah and McClelland (1991), Funnell and Sheridan (1992), and Farah, Meyer, and McMullen (in press). At present it seems that knowledge of living things can be impaired, that the impairment is probably in visual semantics, and that this is a later stage of processing than the visual impairment in prosopagnosia.

The idea that pure alexia is a form of visual agnosia resulting from an impairment in the rapid recognition of multiple shapes, as suggested in section 5.3, has found increasing support over the past few years. Farah and Wallace (1991) summarize the evidence to that date and present new supporting evidence. Further evidence can be found in Behrmann and Shallice (in press).

Finally, the utility of thinking about the effects of brain damage in terms of connectionist networks, which might have been regarded as questionable just five years ago (indeed "questionable" is a nicer word than one prepublication reviewer used!), has been demonstrated many times over in recent years. Starting with the seminal work of Hinton and Shallice (1991), Patterson, Seidenberg, and McClelland (1989), and others, the underlying mechanisms of many neuropsychological syndromes have been illuminated by connectionist modeling. Some connectionist reinterpretations of visual disorders following brain damage, and their implications for theories of normal vision, can be found in Farah (1994a, b) and accompanying commentaries.

Martha J. Farah
Philadelphia, October 1994

References

Behrmann, M., and Shallice, T. (in press). Pure alexia: A nonspatial visual disorder affecting letter activation. *Cognitive Neuropsychology*.

Burton, A. M., Young, A. W., Bruce, V., Johnston, R. A., and Ellis, A. W. (1991). Understanding covert recognition. *Cognition*, 39, 129–166.

De Haan, E. H. F., Bauer, R. M., and Greve, K. W. (1992). Behavioral and physiological evidence for covert recognition in a prosopagnosic patient. *Cortex*, 28, 77–95.

De Renzi, E., Perani, D., Carlesimo, G. A., Silveri, M. C., and Fazio, F. (1994). Prosopagnosia can be associated with damage confined to the right hemisphere—An MRI and PET study and a review of the literature. *Neuropsychologia*, 32, 893–902.

Farah, M. J. (1994a). Neuropsychological inference with an interactive brain: A critique of the "locality assumption." *Behavioral and Brain Sciences*, 17, 43–61.

Farah, M. J. (1994b). Interactions on the interactive brain. *Behavioral and Brain Sciences*, 17, 90–104.

Farah, J. M., Levinson, K. L., and Klein, K. L. (in press). Face recognition and within-category discrimination in prosopagnosia. *Neuropsychologia*.

Farah, M. J., and McClelland, J. L. (1991). A computational model of semantic memory impairment: Modality-specificity and emergent category-specificity. *Journal of Experimental Psychology: General*, 120, 339–357.

Farah, M. J., McMullen, P. A., and Meyer, M. M. (1991). Can recognition of living things be selectively impaired? *Neuropsychologia*, 29, 185–193.

Farah, M. J., Meyer, M. M., and McMullen, P. A. (in press). The living/nonliving dissociation is not an artifact: Giving an a priori implausible hypothesis a strong test. *Cognitive Neuropsychology*.

Farah, M. J., O'Reilly, R. C., and Vecera, S. P. (1993). Dissociated overt and covert recognition as an emergent property of lesioned attractor networks. *Psychological Review*, 100, 571–588.

Farah, M. J. Tanaka, J. W., and Drain, H. M. (in press). What causes the face inversion effect? *Journal of Experimental Psychology: Human Perception and Performance*.

Farah, M. J., and Wallace, M. A. (1991). Pure alexia as a visual impairment: A reconsideration. *Cognitive Neuropsychology*, 8, 313–334.

Farah, M. J., Wilson, K. D., Drain, H. M., and Tanaka, J. W. (in press). The inverted face inversion effect: Evidence for mandatory, face-specific perceptual mechanisms. *Vision Research*.

Feinberg, T. E., Schindler, R. J., Ochoa, R. J., Kwan, P. C., and Farah, M. J. (in press). Associative visual agnosia and alexia without prosopagnosia. *Cortex*.

Funnell, E., and Sheridan, J. (1992). Categories of knowledge? Unfamiliar aspects of living and non-living things. *Cognitive Neuropsychology*, 9, 135–154.

Haxby, J. V., Grady, C. L., Horowitz, B., Ungerleider, L. G., Mishkin, M., Carson, R. E., Herscovitch, P., Schapiro, M. B., and Rapoport, S. I. (1991). Dissociation of object and spatial visual processing pathways in human extrastriate cortex. *Proceedings of the National Academy of Sciences*, 88, 1621–1625.

Hinton, G. E., and Shallice T. (1991). Lesioning an attractor network: Investigations of acquired dyslexia. *Brain*, 98, 96–121.

McNeil, J. E., and Warrington, E. K. (1993). Prosopagnosia: A face-specific disorder. *Quarterly Journal of Experimental Psychology*, 46A, 1–10.

Patterson, K. E., Seidenberg, M. S., and McClelland, J. L. (1989). Connections and disconnections: Acquired dyslexia in a computational model of reading processes. In

R. G. M. Morris (Ed.), *Parallel Distributing Processing: Implications for Psychology and Neurobiology*. New York: Oxford University Press.

Sergent, J., Ohta, S., and MacDonald, B. (1992). Functional neuroanatomy of face and object processing. *Brain*, 115, 15–36.

Sergent, J., Zuck, E., Levesque, M., and MacDonald, B. (1992). Positron emission tomography study of letter and object processing. *Cerebral Cortex*, 2, 68–80.

Tanaka, J. W., and Farah, M. J. (1993). Parts and wholes in face recognition. *Quarterly Journal of Experimental Psychology*, 46A, 225–245.

Name Index

Subject Index